Developing Ocular Motor and Visual Perceptual Skills

An Activity Workbook

Developing Ocular Motor and Visual Perceptual Skills

An Activity Workbook

Kenneth A. Lane, OD, FCOVD
Lane Learning Center
Lewisville, TX

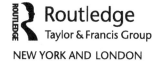

Routledge
Taylor & Francis Group

NEW YORK AND LONDON

Cover art and interior illustrations by Kevin White

First published in 2005 by SLACK Incorporated

Published 2024 by Routledge
605 Third Avenue, New York, NY 10017
4 Park Square, Milton Park, Abingdon, Oxon OX14 4RN

Routledge is an imprint of the Taylor & Francis Group, an informa business

Lane, Kenneth A.
   Developing ocular motor and visual perceptual skills : an activity workbook / Kenneth A. Lane.
      p. ; cm.
   ISBN 1-55642-595-3 (alk. paper)
   1. Vision disorders in children. 2. Eye--Movement disorders. 3. Visual perception in children. 4. Visual training. 5. Learning disabled children.
         [DNLM: 1. Eye Movements--Child. 2. Learning Disorders--rehabilitation--Child. 3. Occupational Therapy--methods--Child. 4. Reading--Child. 5. Visual Perception--Child. WW 400 L265d 2005] I. Title.

RE48.2.C5L358 2005
618.92'0977--dc22
                            2004020420

   ISBN: 9781556425950 (pbk)
   ISBN: 9781003523819 (ebk)

   DOI: 10.4324/9781003523819

Dedication

Dedicated to my father, Howard S. Lane.

Contents

OM-1 Colored Overlays
OM-2 Figure Ground
OM-3 Static Fixation
OM-4 Line Counting
OM-5 Fixation Activities
OM-6 Four Corner Fixation
OM-7 Pencil Pursuits
OM-8 Number Pursuits
OM-9 Global Scanning
OM-10 Letter Search
OM-11 Words in Words
OM-12 Visual Scanning
OM-13 Yardstick Fixations
OM-14 Pencils With Numbers
OM-15 String Reading
OM-16 Near-Far Letter Naming
OM-17 Baseball Fixations
OM-18 Spatial Attention
OM-19 Peripheral Training
OM-20 Marsden Ball
OM-21 VMC Bat
OM-22 Brock String
OM-23 Pursuit Reading
OM-24 Dictionary Training
OM-25 Board–Book Reading
OM-26 Orthography Activities

GM-1 One Foot Hop
GM-2 Stepping Stones
GM-3 Heel and Toe Rock
GM-4 Pattern Hopping
GM-5 Gross Motor Balance Sequencing
GM-6 Foot Tapping
GM-7 Bean Bag Basketball
GM-8 Crawling Activities
GM-9 Marine Crawl
GM-10 Creeping Activities

Acknowledgments

This book would never have been completed without the help of these individuals:

Special thanks to Bob Williams and Vision Extension, Inc., for letting me use and revise activities from my first book, *Reversal Errors: Theories and Therapy Procedures*.

To Vicki Neville, who spent countless hours typing and helping to organize this book.

To Kevin White, for his advice, cover design, and the artwork used throughout this book.

To Judi Bowman and Kathy McDaniel, for proofreading.

Special thanks to SLACK Incorporated, for giving me the opportunity to write this book.

Preface

My years of working with school-aged children have shown me that many children who are experiencing learning difficulties in school can be helped, especially if help is given at an early age. Young children who are reversing letters and numbers, who have poor printing skills, or are having difficulty learning to read are often immature in the basic perceptual and motor skills needed to do these tasks. Waiting and hoping that they will outgrow these difficulties is not advisable. Many children never totally overcome these difficulties, which can affect their self-esteem the rest of their lives.

This book is designed so that optometrists and occupational therapists, as well as parents and teachers, can help children to avoid school failure. This book does not teach children to read. However, it gives a child the skills that make it easier for him to be taught.

My background as a developmental optometrist has given me the unique opportunity to look at a child's learning difficulties through the eyes of someone who has extensive knowledge of the visual system. Developmental optometrists believe that by improving the efficiency of a child's or adult's visual system, you can improve their quality of life. They believe that since vision is learned, it can be enhanced through visual training activities. Visual training is a sequence of activities to develop efficient visual skills and visual processing. Effective training requires visual skills to be developed until they are integrated with other systems and become automatic. Some visual training activities require the use of lenses, prisms, filters, occluders, and other specialized instruments, and can only be administered under the guidance of an optometrist. However, the activities in this book do not require specialized equipment and can be administered by anyone.

I learned very early in my career that learning disabilities are often caused by multiple problems. There is no single cause, and therefore, I knew vision was not the whole answer. Reading the work of Jean Ayres on sensory integration seemed to fill the void. Sensory integration is the neurological process that organizes sensation from one's own body and from the environment and makes it possible to use the body effectively within the environment. The spatial and temporal aspects of inputs from different sensory modalities are interpreted, associated, and unified. Sensory integration is information processing (Fisher, 1991).

I decided to write a book that incorporates the best of sensory integration and vision therapy so that the child receives the best from both worlds. I also used the following theories to develop the activities.

1. New research in the cerebellum gave me the ideas for some of the activities, especially activities that deal with sequencing.
2. Dual vision processing theories gave me ideas of how to improve visual scanning.
3. Harold Levinson's theories on cerebellum-vestibular dysfunction gave me ideas for visual motor and eye tracking.
4. Piaget's theories on the child's conception of space helped me to develop activities for visual motor activities.
5. Keith Rayner's theories on eye movements and reading gave me ideas for eye tracking training.

I urge those who want to learn more about the American Optometric Association's description of vision therapy to read *Vision, Learning, and Dyslexia: A Joint Organizational Policy Statement of the American Academy of Optometry and the American Optometric Association* (American Optometric Association, 1997). In addition to this, *The Occupational Therapy Practice Framework: Domain and Process* was designed to articulate occupational therapy's focus and actions (AOTA, 2002).

Throughout this book, I use the pronouns, "he" and "him" to denote children. This is not intended to discriminate against females or to insinuate that only males need help in these areas. This is used solely for simplicity in the grammatical construction of the text.

I urge occupational therapists who feel that the child with whom they are working may have a serious vision problem to seek help with a developmental optometrist in their area. A developmental optometrist specializes in vision training procedures and is qualified to evaluated children with learning disabilities. The main body of developmental optometrists is the College of Optometrists in Vision Development (COVD). This group has its main office in St. Louis, MO (see Appendix) and offers a fellowship program that requires written and oral testing to verify competency. Likewise, if an optometrist feels that the child needs additional occupational therapy, he should see an occupational therapist in his area. We all need to work together to give these children the help they need and deserve.

All children should have a complete visual evaluation by an optometrist before they start the activities in this book. I have included important names and addresses in the Appendix B to be used to locate qualified help.

References

American Occupational Therapy Association. The occupational therapy practice framework: Domain & process. *Amer J Occup Ther*, 2002, 609-639.

American Optometric Association (1997). Vision, learning and dyslexia. A joint organizational policy statement of the American Academy of Optometry and the American Optometric Association. *Journal of Optometric Vision Development*, 56, 98-100.

Fisher, A. G. (1991). *Sensory integration: Theory and practice.* Philadelphia, PA: F. A. Davis Company.

Chapter One

HOW TO USE THIS BOOK

The activities in this book are designed to help give a child the necessary skills needed to succeed in school. The activities are divided into the following categories:

1. Ocular Motor
2. Gross Motor
3. Visual-Motor Perception
4. Visual Memory
5. Laterality
6. Reversals

The activities in each category are not in any particular order. All activities are of equal importance. You do not have to start with the first activity in each category. Use the questionnaire in the Appendix to give to the parents to help you determine which categories to use. The chapters preceding the activities will give you tips on the best way to proceed in each category of activities. Each activity is divided into levels of difficulty with Level 1 being the easiest and Level 5 being the most difficult. Level 1 is designed for children with developmental ages of 4 through 5. Level 2 is for children 6 years old, Level 3 for 7-year-olds, Level 4 for 8-year-olds, and Level 5 for age 9 and above. Remember, there is a difference between developmental and chronological age. You will need to test or estimate the child's developmental age. For example, if you have a 6-year-old child with very poor motor skills, you will probably start at Level 1. If you have no idea where to start, start at Level 1. If it is too easy, then go to Level 2. The idea is not to start with too difficult an activity. You don't want to frustrate the child or create feelings of low self-esteem. Once you start working with a child, you will get a feeling as to where to start. Some activities don't start at Level 1. In those cases, I did not feel the activity was appropriate for a 4- or 5-year-old, so the lowest level listed is where I want you to start.

There are hundreds of activities in this book. Have the child experience as many as possible; however, you may need to spend more time in one category than another. If you have a child with very poor gross motor skills, you may want to do more activities in this area than laterality, for example.

In order for the activities to be beneficial, it is recommended that a child work on them three times a week. The suggested number of activities per session is five, with the time allotted for each activity to be 10 minutes. The length of time and the number of activities can vary depending on the time available and the child's ability to attend to a task. If a child is getting a lot of benefit from one activity, then continue with that activity at the next therapy session; however, do not do the same activity more than six sessions in a row. Make a note of a particular beneficial activity and go back to it again at a later date. Learn how to vary and mix the activities. For example, you don't want to do all gross motor activities at one session. By varying the activities, you will keep the child's interest and have a more successful program.

If an activity is too difficult for the child, go down to the next lowest level. If there is no lower level, then do another activity. For example, if the child is having a lot of difficulty with one visual motor activity, try another visual motor activity.

To summarize:

1. Do at least five activities per session for at least 10 minutes each.
2. Vary the categories to get a good mix.
3. Start at Level 1 for children 5 and under.
4. If an activity is too difficult, go the next lowest level. If there is no lower level, do another activity in the same category.
5. Activities that are too difficult can be repeated at a later date.
6. If an activity is too easy, go to the next highest level.
7. Stay with an activity until you feel the child has mastered it, but try not to do the same activity more than six times in a row. Make a note and repeat it later.
8. Use the questionnaire in the Appendix to help you determine what categories to use. The underlined category is the main category for a particular problem. Do more activities from this category.

Each activity is numbered; for example, all the laterality activities start with an "L" and the gross motor activities start with "GM".

An example of a daily lesson plan would be:

GM-1, Level 1
GM-4, Level 2
VM-1 Level 2
OM-1, Level 1
VM-2, Level 1

This means that on this day, the child will do two gross motor activities. They are: Gross Motor 1/Level 1 and Gross Motor 4/Level 2. Also, they would do Visual Motor 1/Level 2, Ocular Motor 1/Level 1, and Visual Memory 2/Level 1. Remember to look at the tips at the end of each chapter. This will help you in designing your lesson plans. In the beginning, try to have a motor activity in each lesson plan. If a child has severe ocular motor problems, you will probably want to do at least two ocular motor activities. If there is a severe reversal problem, you may need to do two reversal activities. Children often have a combination of problems and usually will have difficulties in all areas. In this case, vary your lesson plans. For example, have two ocular motor activities one day and two gross motor activities the next day.

The secrets of having a good activities program are:

1. Have a good understanding of why a certain activity is beneficial for the child.

2. Have a good understanding of the child's developmental age.

3. Move quickly from activity to activity because often children have very short attention spans.

4. Know how to vary the activities to benefit the child the most.

5. Keep a good record of what activities have been previously given and take good notes of your observations.

6. Develop a good rapport with the child, and most of all, keep the activities fun so the child does not become bored after a few weeks. This is done by constantly varying the activities.

We have to remember that we are not teaching a child to read. We are giving him the skills to make learning easier.

There is nothing more satisfying than to see a child who has been struggling in school and feels that he is inferior to start to enjoy reading and develop a good self-image. We are lucky because we see this happen on a daily basis.

Chapter Two

THE COMPLEXITY
OF READING

Reading is the most complex and intriguing skill that has evolved in the human race. (Mason, 1975)

We all take reading for granted because it is automatic for most of us; however, for many children, it is a nightmare. Reading is the most complex and intriguing skill that has evolved in the human race (Mason, 1975). It involves serial and parallel stages of visual processing, sensorimotor coordination, and cognitive and linguistic processing (Garzia, 1996). Between 2% and 20% of the US school population have some type of reading disorder.

Why is reading so difficult for some children? In order to try to understand this, we have to look at several areas. These areas include: the difference between spoken and written language, the human brain, the history of reading, the complexity of reading, and especially English and society's emphasis on reading.

Whereas speaking is natural, reading is not. We are given years to learn to speak but only months to learn to read. Unlike speaking, reading is not an instinctive human ability. There isn't a reading center in the brain (D'Arcangelo, 1999). However, there is a speaking center. Language is localized to a broad central wedge of the left hemisphere known as the perisylvian cortex (for the way it surrounds the Sylvian fissure, the deep horizontal canyon that separates the temporal from the frontal and parietal lobes). The processing of language is much more complicated than was originally thought. For example, recent data now suggests that the language areas of the brain are divided by semantics and syntax. The left posterior areas are activated during tasks involving the meaning of words, while the left frontal cortex is more specifically activated during tasks involving grammatical processing. For instance, Boca's area lights up when subjects compare two sentences whose meaning is identical but that differ in the order of their words—that is syntactic structure. On the other hand, the left temporal-parietal area (including Wernicke's area as well as a large area above and behind it) is turned on more by tasks that tax one's understanding of individual words, like hearing the anomalous sentence "We bake cookies in the zoo". In other words, the posterior language center is the place where the meanings of words is stored, like a mental dictionary, and the frontal center functions like a grammar textbook. To make this even more complicated, nouns are retrieved in the left temporal parietal region, while verbs are processed in the frontal lobe (Eliot, 1999) (Figure 2-1).

When a person reads, there is stimulation in the back of the brain that includes the occipital region, which is activated by the visual features of the letters, the angular gyrus, where print is transcribed into language, and Wernickes region, which accesses meaning.

As you can see, the neurological processes of reading and language are extremely complex. You would think that with something as complex as reading, we would give our children adequate time to learn it, but this does not appear to be the case. School pressures and work expected of children today are much more intense than they used to be. Children who graduate from kindergarten today are expected to be able to know their letter and blend sounds and recognize some words. There is no doubt that we are pushing some of these children too fast. Many children are not mature enough to handle the complex process of reading. This becomes apparent when we compare our incidence of learning disabilities in the US to the children in Europe. Europeans exhibit a low incidence of learning disabilities because they do not begin their children's reading training until they are 7 to 9 years old (Weimer, 2000).

In order to get a better understanding of the complex nature of reading, we need to have a better understanding of the intricate nature of the human brain and its development. The brain weighs about 3 pounds, just two percent of the total weight of a 150-pound person, but uses between 20 to 25% of the body's oxygen and a substantial amount of calories we consume in the form of blood sugar (glucose). Each brain signal is measured in millivolts. In total, the brain generates about 20 watts of power at any given time. The typical brain has 100 billion neurons, each connected to 1000 or more other neurons (Fauber, 2002). A neuron takes a million times longer to send a signal than a typical computer switch. Yet the brain can recognize a familiar face in less than a second, a feat beyond the ability of the most powerful computers. The brain achieves this speed because unlike the step by step computer, its billions of neurons can all attack the problem simultaneously (Allman, 1988). In other words, we think with our whole brain and read and solve complex problems with our whole brain. This is why it is important for us to do activities that involve the whole brain.

The process of brain development begins during the first month of gestation and is far from complete at birth. The necessary 100 billion nerve cells are installed at birth but most aren't connected (Muha, 1999). At birth, a child's cerebral cortex has all the neurons that it will ever have. In fact, the brain produces an overabundance of neurons, nearly twice as many as it will need. Beginning at about 28 weeks of prenatal development, a massive pruning of neurons begins, resulting in a loss of 1/3 to 1/2 of these elements. While the brain is pruning away excess neurons, a tremendous increase in dendrites adds substantially to the surface area available for synapses (the functional connections among cells). At the fastest rate, connections are built at the incredible speed of 3 billion per second. During the period of birth to age 10, the number of synaptic connections continues to rise rapidly, then begins to drop and continues to decline slowly into adult life (Wolfe, 1998). The brain remains highly plastic and capable of extensive neural reorganization throughout life. Even though there are critical periods, we can con-

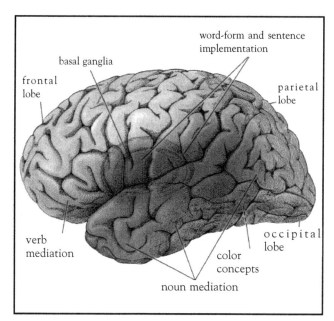

Figure 2-1. Functions of the brain.

tinue to learn throughout life. The brain requires certain levels of stimuli, such as touch, speech, and images to be present for complete, normal development (Bruer, 1998).

It is interesting to note that the early years, which are most crucial for learning, receive the least emphasis in federal, state, and local programs. The US government spends at least seven times more on the elderly than on children from birth to age 5 (Wolfe, 1998).

As you have discovered by now, reading is obviously a very complex task, and as with all things, there is a history behind it. If you compressed the history of life on earth into 24 hours, multicellular organisms appeared in the last 12 hours, dinosaurs in the last 4, the earliest man in the last 40 seconds, and modern man less than a second ago. It has taken 2 billion years for primitive cells to incorporate a nucleus, but only 200 million years (1/10 of that time) to evolve multicellular animals and 4 million years to go from small brained apes with crude bone tools to modern man (Crichton, 2002). A vocal tract capable of producing the sounds to articulate speech had been developed among humans 600,000 years before we have any independent evidence that our forebears were using language or speaking (100,000 years ago) (Tattersall, 2001). The first writing by Sumerians of Mesopotamia occurred about 3000 BC. This is about the same time as the invention of the wheel. Alphabets started in modern Syria during the second millennium BC. All new existing alphabets were ultimately derived from that ancestral Semitic alphabet (Diamond, 1999). By 400 AD, the classical scroll had been all but abandoned and most books were being produced as gathered leaves in a rectangular format. They were then folded several times. By the sixteenth

century, the formats of folded sheets had become official. Between 1450 and 1455, Gutenberg produced a bible with 42 lines to each page. This was the first book ever printed from type (Manguel, 1996). As you can see, in a mere 250 generations, we have gone from the first written word to where we are now. This in itself is interesting, but also consider that it is only recently that all classes of people have had the opportunity to learn to read. Well into the middle ages, writers assumed that their readers would hear rather than see the text. Since few people could read, there were public readings. Medieval texts repeatedly call upon the audience to "lend ears" (Manguel, 1996). Therefore, unlike speech, reading is a very new process.

The difficulty with reading is worsened when you consider the complexity of English. English is not easy because of the abstract nature of phonemes (especially consonants) and the fact that most alphabets do not code each vowel with a unique symbol. Regarding the first issue, young children often have an imperfect idea of what phonemes are because they are abstractions rather than natural physical segments of speech. For example, the vowel sound "bat" is about the same as the one in "laugh" and because both vowels tend to have a relatively long duration, in both words, the sound can be clearly heard. Thus, the teacher can point to the a in "bat" and the child can hear the vowel sound clearly, because it has sufficient duration no matter which sound precedes it. In contrast, the pronunciation of a consonant can be highly dependent on the vowels that precede and follow it. For example, the d in "dime" is different acoustically from the d in "lid". Regarding the second issue, English does not code each vowel sound with a unique symbol. English has more than a dozen vowel sounds but only five standard vowel letters (Rayne, 2001). It has 1120 different ways of spelling its 40 phonemes (the sound required to pronounce all its words). If "tongue" is pronounced "tung", why isn't "argue" pronounced "arg"; and if "enough" is pronounced "enuff", why isn't "bough" pronounced "buff" (Kher, 2001)?

Processes involved in reading include *syntax*, which is the knowledge of grammar and word associations to make sense of a sentence; *semantics*, which is knowledge of word meaning; and *context clues*, which is using the familiarity of the topic to help in word identification. Good readers also are able to use their knowledge of spelling patterns (orthography) to help in letter identification. In the English language, letters occur in certain positions in words more frequently than in other positions (Mayzner & Tresselt, 1965). For example, in the pseudo-word "hortey", all the letters are in positions they are normally in for a six letter English word. In the pseudo-word "yterho", all the letters are not in position they are normally in for a six letter word. As you can see, hortey is much easier to pronounce and remember than yterho (Wicklund &

Katz, 1977). By being in positions they are normally in, the letters help to identify each other just as words help to identify each other in sentences because they are in positions they are normally in. Good readers use this knowledge for letter identification when they don't have enough feature detectors for normal identification.

Learning to read is an amazing accomplishment. Many famous people have had a great deal of difficulty learning to read, including the poet W. B. Yeats and the artist Leonardo da Vinci (Kher, 2001). Thomas Edison also had difficulty with reading. He said, "I remember I used to never be able to get along at school. I was always at the foot of the class. I used to feel that the teachers did not sympathize with me and my father thought I was stupid". The following is a letter that Thomas Edison (his family called him Al) wrote to his mother:

Dear Mother:

Started the store several weeks I have growed considerably I don't look much like a boy now - Hows all the foks did you receive a box of Books from Memphis that he promised to send them - languages

Your son Al (Aaron, 1988)

Many people have overcome their reading difficulties. The difference between those individuals and others is their self-image. If a child feels good about himself, he will succeed. If he feels that he is inferior, he will fail. This is why we must identify and help these children at an early age.

Many children have difficulty learning to read and they are often labeled. The most common label you will hear is *dyslexia*. Dyslexia is a term implying impairment in reading. The prefix "dys" is from Latin meaning bad. The root "lexia" is Greek and relates to speech (Griffin, 1999). Dyslexia was first termed by British ophthalmologists and was considered to be a visual problem. In 1930, Dr. Samuel Orton, a physician, stated it was from mixed dominance. In the 1950s and 1960s, it was thought to be perceptual deficiencies. Since then, the visual and perceptual theories have been replaced by theories dealing with a lack of phonemic awareness (Rumsey, 1992). It seems strange that a lack of phonemic awareness is the main cause of developmental dyslexia when it is rarely the cause for acquired dyslexia. This makes you wonder why the visual and perceptual theories are now almost completely ignored by many professionals. People need to keep an open mind on the subject. I feel that it is probably a combination of all three.

The World Federation of Neurology says dyslexia is a disorder manifested by difficulty learning to read despite conventional instruction, adequate intelligence, and sociocultural opportunity (Estes, 1989). It is dependent upon fundamental and cognitive disabilities, which are frequently of constitutional origin. Most theoreticians state that 3% to 6% of school-aged children are dyslexic (Estes,

1989). Dyslexia is the bottom end of the reading scale. As stated earlier, up to 20% of school aged children have severe difficulty in learning to read. Only the lower 3% to 6% are dyslexic. The other 14% to 17% have a learning disability (LD). The definition of a learning disability is the same as dyslexia; however, these children are not as severely affected. True dyslexia is fairly rare; however, the term is greatly overused by our school systems and is mainly used to help children qualify for extra help. There is no known cause or cure for dyslexia. A child who suddenly starts to have reading problems in third grade and did well in grades kindergarten through second is not dyslexic. A dyslexic child will have learning difficulties from kindergarten through adult life.

Dyslexia is an inability to read words accurately. My experience has shown that there are as many female as male dyslexics. Twenty to 40% of these children also have an attention disorder. Thirty-five to 40% of boys and 17% to 18% of girls have a parent with dyslexia (Rumsey, 1992). Dyslexic problems include:

1. Poor coordination.
2. Poor spatial reasoning.
3. Right-left directional confusion.
4. Poor temporal orientation.
5. Poor color naming.
6. Mixed cerebral dominance.
7. Linear tracking errors (Council on Scientific Affairs, 1989).
8. Ninety-two percent of dyslexics have poor ocular motor skills.
9. Eighty-three percent have poor hand-eye tracking.
10. Ninety-eight percent have poor visual-motor integration coordination (Blythe, 2001).
11. They have a large number of regressive eye movements when they read (Punnett, 1984).

There are three types of dyslexia:

1. *Dyseidesia dyslexia*: The child has difficulty with whole words and tends to write words with phonetic spelling.
2. *Dysphonesia dyslexia*: The child has trouble using phonics to decode the word. He either knows it by "look say" or not at all.
3. *Dysphoneidesia dyslexia*: The child has characteristics of both (Griffin, 1992).

Researchers have been trying to find the cause of dyslexia since the term was first used in 1887 (Shaywitz, 1987). We have a good idea of the areas of the brain involved and we know from brain scans that dyslexic children have to use four times as much lactic acid in the sound processing portions of the brain compared to normal readers (*Charlotte Observer*, 2000). This shows they have to exert four times the effort to read compared to normal children. There is no single theory that describes the cause of dyslexia. The following are the current theories on dyslexia.

1. *Phonological Deficit Hypothesis*: This has been the dominant explanatory framework for dyslexia. It argues that neurological abnormalities in the language areas around the Sylvian fissure lead to failure to develop phonological awareness skills at the age of 5, thereby interfering with the learning of phoneme-grapheme and grapheme-phoneme conversions, which are critical requirements in learning to read. There is evidence that phonological awareness deficits persist through life.

2. *Magnocellular Deficit Hypothesis*: Like children with language disorders, children with dyslexia take longer to process rapidly changing auditory stimuli. Neuroanatomical abnormalities have been identified in both the visual and auditory magnocellular pathways to the thalamus. Visual magnocellular pathways abnormalities may cause visual persistence, which would lead to specific difficulties in reading. It has been suggested that magnocellular abnormalities may lead to difficulties in most types of rapid processing. Chapter Four explains this theory in detail.

3. *Double Deficit Theory*: This theory states that phonological deficit and naming speed deficits represent two separable sources of reading dysfunction and that developmental dyslexia is characterized by both phonological and naming speed "core" deficits. Dyslexic children are slow at saying the names of pictures or colors. They are also slower in their choice reaction to an auditory tone or a flash of light in complete absence of phonological task components.

4. *Cerebellar Deficit Hypothesis*: Dyslexics show a wide range of deficits. These include: balance, motor skills, phonological skills, and rapid processing. Children with dyslexia suffer problems in fluency for any skill that should become automatic via extensive practice. Deficits in motor skills and automalization point strongly to the cerebellum. There is clear evidence that the cerebellum is involved in reading. A cerebellar deficit, therefore, provides one explanation of the range of problems suffered by children with dyslexia (Fawcett, 2001). This theory is explained in greater detail in Chapter Five.

We need to have a clear understanding of both the Cerebellar Deficit Hypothesis and the Magnocellular Deficit Hypothesis. Most of the activities in this book are based on these two theories. Most remediation today on dyslexia is based on the Phonological Deficit Hypothesis. Phonological training by itself is no more the answer for dyslexia than any other theory is by itself. Dyslexic children need more than phonics. We can give these children the help that the school systems cannot give. By identifying children who are at risk early and having them do the activities in the book, we can keep children from experiencing school failure and developing a low self-esteem that can affect them the rest of their lives. The following are symptoms of children who are at risk for school difficulties:

1. Delayed speech or motor development, or has had speech therapy.

2. Poor gross motor skills.

3. Very poor and disorganized visual motor skills.

4. Birth complications or a birth weight under 5 pounds.

5. Poor ability to pay attention or concentrate in a boring situation.

6. Father or mother who had learning difficulties.

7. Excessive reversing of letters or numbers.

8. Difficulty learning his alphabet.

9. Difficulty with letter and number recognition.

10. Makes mistakes copying from the board or his textbook.

11. Skips words or loses his place easily when he reads.

Reading requires a multitude of skills. Not only must the brain move the eyes to the proper location, but the visual image must focus on the fovea. The letter's visual features, orientation, and position in the word must be interpreted and coded. This information plus knowledge of orthography, syntax, semantics, context, and peripheral visual clues are all used to help identify the word. Adult readers have the luxury of using all of this information when they read. Young readers, however, do not. Consider the fact that a good reader in first grade only looks at about 30% of a word for each fixation (Morris, 1973). That is not much more than one or two letters at a time. This indicates that young children spend most of their reading time decoding individual letters and letter groups to form words. Basic perceptual skills are absolutely necessary for the young child to succeed in reading. Perceptual skills are needed to break down the visual image and code the individual prerequisites such as feature identification, letter orientation, and proper sequencing. They must also have the visual skills necessary for proper focusing on the individual letters and the fine motor skills necessary for proper and accurate eye movements.

The purpose of this chapter is to give you a better understanding of the complex processes involved in reading. With this new understanding, you will be better equipped with the skills to assist the child who is struggling in school and give him optimum opportunity to achieve success throughout his school years and life.

References

Aaron, P. G. (1988). Specific reading disability in historically famous persons. *Journal of Learning Disabilities, 21.*

Allman, W. F. (1988). How the brain really works its wonders. *U.S. News and World Report, 104,* 48(6).

Blythe, S. G. (2001). Neurological dysfunction as a significant factor in children with dyslexia. *Journal of Behavioral Optometry, 12*(6), 145.

Bruer, J. T. (1998). Brain science, brain fiction. *Educational Leadership, 56*(3), 14-18.

Council on Scientific Affairs, American Medical Association. (1989). Dyslexia. *JAMA, 261*(15), 2236.

Crichton, M. (2002). *Prey.* Harper-Collins Publishers.

D'Arcangelo, M. (1999). Learning about learning to read: A conversation with Sally Shaywitz. *Educational Leadership, 57,* 26-31.

Diamond, J. (1999). *Guns, germs, and steel.* New York: W. W. Norton and Company.

Eliot, L. (1999). *What's going on in there?* New York: Bantam Books.

Estes, H. E. (1989). Dyslexia (council report). *JAMA, 261,* 2236-2239.

Fauber, J. (2002). Work on the brain gives scientists more insight into human body. *Milwaukee Journal Sentinel.*

Fawcett, A. J. (2001). Cerebellar tests differentiate between groups of poor readers with and without IQ discrepancy. *Journal of Learning Disabilities, 34*(2), 119.

Garzia, R. P. (1996). Vision and reading II. *Journal of Optometric Vision Development, 194,* 25, 4-26.

Griffin, J. R. (1999). Optometry's role in reading dysfunction. *Optometric Vision Development, 30*(3), 122-131.

Griffin, J. R. (1992). Prevalence of dyslexia. *Journal of Optometric Vision Development, 23,* 17-22.

Kher, U. (2001). Blame it on the written word. *Time, 56.*

Manguel, A. (1996). *A history of reading.* New York: Penguin.

Mason, M. (1975). Reading ability and letter search time. *Journal of Experimental Psychology, 104:* 146-166.

Mayzner, M. S., Tresselt, M. E. (1965). Tables of single-letter and diagram frequency counts for various word-length and letter position combinations. *Psychonomic Press, 1*(2).

Morris, H. F. (1973). *Manual for the edl/biometris reading eye II.* New York: McGraw-Hill, Inc.

Muha, L. (1999). Your baby's amazing brain. *Parenting,* 8A, 40-45.

New method turns dyslexic teens into readers. (2000). *Charlotte Observer.*

Punnett, A. F. (1984). Relationship between reinforcement and eye movements during ocular motor training with learning disabled children. *Journal of Learning Disabilities, 17*(1), 16-19.

Rayne, K. (2001). How psychological science informs the teaching of reading. *Journal of the American Psychological Society, 2*(2), 31-74.

Rumsey, J. M. (1992). The biology of developmental dyslexia. *JAMA,* V268, 912.

Shaywitz, B. A. (1987). Dyslexia (editorial). *The New England Journal of Medicine, 316*(20), 1268-1270.

Tattersall, I. (2001). How we came to be human. *Scientific American,* 56-63.

Weimer, L. (2000). Helping kids' coordination, self-esteem. *San Jose Mercury News.*

Wicklund, D. A., & Katz, L. (1977). Perception and retention in children's reading, COVD, Paper Number 160981, Connecticut University Department of Psychology.

Wolfe, P. (1998). What do we know from brain research? *Educational Leadership, 56*(3), 8-13.

Chapter Three

EYE MOVEMENTS AND READING

"The control of eye movements during reading can be considered to involve temporal and spatial decisions." (Rayner, 1983)

Introduction

This chapter is one of the most important chapters in this book. You must have a clear understanding on how ocular motor exercises help a child with reading difficulties. This requires a good knowledge of eye movements and reading.

We have already discussed the complexity of the human brain. It is staggering to think that the cerebral cortex alone has about 10 billion neurons and 1 million billion connections or synapses. Counting one synapse per second, we would finish counting 32 million years from now. If we consider the number of ways in which circuits or loops of connections would be stimulated, we would be dealing with a 10 followed by at least a million zeros. There are 10 followed by 79 zeros, give or take a few, particles in the known universe (Edelman, 1998). Considering how complex the brain is, one of its most complex assignments is reading and one of the most important parts of reading is moving the eyes across the page of print in perfect harmony to be able to encode print. Encoding enables the brain to form a visual or non-visual code of the word and place it in working memory (Krueger, 1993). In decoding, the letter components are accessed and compared against target letters in memory and the word is remembered.

It is important to remember that the brain can't handle all the visual information available to it. Three-quarters of the visual information available to the brain when we read is ignored (Smith, 1994). When we read, we don't take in large amounts of visual information. The eyes move across the page in a series of quick movements called *saccades* and pause to take in visual information called *fixations* (Figure 3-1) (Ygge, 1994). Because only a small fraction of the retina has heightened acuity, the point of fixation must constantly be moved about to allow detailed visual processing. Moreover, this must be done so that each change of gaze places the eye at convenient locations on the target (words). For example, in reading, the eyes must accurately jump from word to word so that when each item is fixated, it can be processed rapidly and the next eye movement can be planned. This requires that each individual eye movement be guided by detailed visual information obtained from locations peripheral to the current point of fixation (Moore, 1999). As I mentioned before, we do not take in a large amount of words as we move our eyes across the line of print (Figures 3-1 and 3-2). The average good reader does not look at more than one word per fixation until he is in the tenth grade (Morris, 1973). Even college students don't take in more than 1.11 words per fixation. A child in first grade only takes in about 45% of a word (Vogel, 1995). The amount of visual information available to the brain during the fixation is called the *perceptual span* or the *span of recognition*.

The perceptual span is the region around the center of vision within which some aspect of visual detail of interest is used in reading (Rayner, 1983). The perceptual span for letter information in words lies asymmetric with respect to the fixation point and extends farther to the right than the left. For Israeli readers, it is the opposite (Rayner, 1983). A skilled reader has an average perceptual span of four characters to the left of fixation and 15 characters to the right (Solan, 2001). Word recognition and processing for comprehension occurs only seven to eight characters to the right of fixation. Information from eight to 15 characters to the right of fixation helps to direct subsequent saccades (Vogel, 1995). While the central foveal areas are processing information for word recognition, parafoveal (peripheral) retinal areas and their corresponding cerebral centers are analyzing word shape and length information to help direct subsequent saccades (Vogel, 1995). Regressive eye movements during reading occur 15% of the time. These are eye movements in the opposite direction (to the left). Most are only a few characters and typically reflect some text confusion or comprehension problem, or perhaps a "recheck" or "double check" confirmation. Children learning to read and poor readers make excessive numbers of regressions (Figure 3-3). Normally, approximately 10% to 15% of all saccades (or fixations) are actually regressive in nature. Uncommon words are refixated more than common words (Ciuffreda, 1995). The average first grader makes 52 regressions per 100 words, while the average college student only makes 15 (Vogel, 1995).

When we pause to take in information as we read, this is called a fixation. The average child in first grade pauses 224 times per 100 words, while the average college student pauses 90 times per 100 words. The average first grader has an average fixation time of .33 seconds, while the average college student pauses for .24 seconds (Vogel, 1995). Because of this, the limit that most people can read is 250 words per minute or about four words per second (Smith 1994). In normal reading, fixations average about 250 msec. During this short interval, visual information is extracted from the printed material (Lovegrove, 1990). Fixation durations are influenced by properties of the text such as word length (Hoffman, 1995). Other factors that can influence longer fixation durations include: low-frequency words, technical words, shorter words, certain grammatical elements, words at the beginning of a new line, words that are misspelled, and regions of the text with important information. Shorter durations of fixation are often caused by the final word of a line, fixations before a regression, and in regions between sentences (Garzia, 1994). The brain is very busy during the fixation. Not only must it encode information but it must decide when to move the eyes and how far to move them for the next fixation. To give you an idea of what happens during

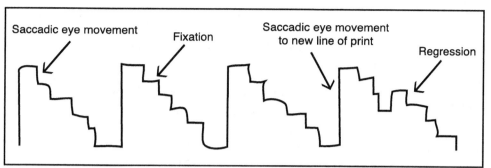

Figure 3-1. The eyes move across the page in a series of quick movements called *saccades* and pause to take in visual information called *fixations*.

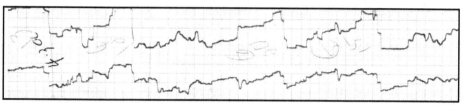

Figure 3-2. We do not take in a large amount of words as we move our eyes across the line of print.

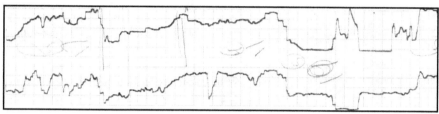

Figure 3-3. Children learning to read and poor readers make excessive numbers of regressions.

the fixation, let's suppose the fixation lasts for 250 msec. We know that much of the visual information necessary for reading can be acquired beginning at about 50 msec into the fixation (Vogel, 1995), leaving the remainder of the fixation (200 msec) to complete programming the next eye movement and for higher level linguistic processing (Rayner, 1983). Processing of information available during the fixation is not completed by the end of the fixation and the onset of the next fixation is not triggered by the completion of processing of information (Rayner, 1983). In other words, the visual processing might be completed but the brain is still digesting information from one fixation to the next fixation. Language aspects of the text must begin having their influence on processing within about 100 msec after the onset of the fixation. This is called *textual influence threshold*. By about 100 msec, the brain has an idea when the next saccade will start, and after 100 msec stimulus changes will not affect when the next saccade will start. This is called the *saccade deadline*. The time when the brain centers have become fully committed to the time of the next saccade is called *the point of no return*, and is estimated to occur at about 30 msec prior to the saccade onset (Rayner, 1983). Contrary to what some people think, all the visual information available to the foveal area is scanned and processed. Good readers do not skip over parts of words when they read. If one letter in a child's foveal vision is masked, his reading speed decreases by 50% (Stanovich, 1993). Children must be taught to scan each letter in a word and every word when they read.

We know that during the fixation the time of the next saccade is determined, but how does the brain know how far to move the eyes for the next fixation? The brain uses a combination of peripheral visual information and knowledge of language patterns to know how far to move the eyes (Rayner, 1983). Visual information such as word length patterns is acquired at least 12 to 15 character positions to the right of the fixation point and specific letter and word shape information no further than 10 character positions to the right of the fixation point (Evans, 1990). There is an optimal landing position for the eyes within a word (Fischer, 1993). The most likely landing spot is near the center of a word. In fact, the location tends to be between the middle and beginning of the word. The preferred viewing location in a five letter word is the second letter and for a ten letter word, it is the fourth (Rayner, 1983). The fixation is less likely to be of the word "the" or on a blank area (Garzia, 1994). If the eyes miss the optimal landing location in the word, the penalty is in the order of 20 msec slower reading speed for every letter that the reader is away from his optimal location (Richman, 1992). Accuracy in saccadic eye movement is obviously a very important component in reading.

Laboratory studies have shown that after the presentation of a visual stimulus, the stimulus continues to be "seen" for some time. The visual response to a stimulus

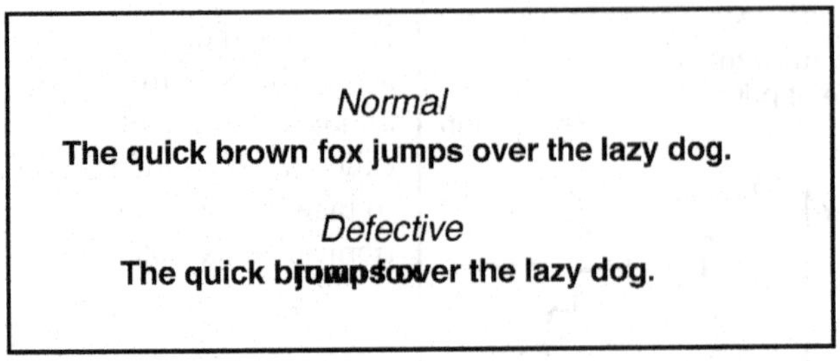

Normal
The quick brown fox jumps over the lazy dog.

Defective
The quick bjompsover the lazy dog.

Figure 3-4. Visual information from one fixation smears into the next fixation like an after image, making the text appear superimposed or overlapping.

outlasts the actual duration of the stimulus. This continuation of a response after the removal of a stimulus is known as visible persistence and can last up to 300 msec. (Lovegrove, 1990). As you can imagine, if this happened when we read, it would cause considerable problems. The brain cannot allow the visual image of one fixation to continue into the next. If this occurred, the two individual visual inputs may be seen but we would not know which was from the first fixation and which was from the second fixation (Lovegrove, 1990). This, of course, does not happen with most readers. However, what does the brain do to overcome this? The answer is that there are two parallel visual subsystems that operate from the retina to the visual cortex. One is called the transient (M cells) and the other is called the sustained (P cells) system.

Retinal images are sampled twice by the visual system (Solan, 1994). It is sampled first by our peripheral vision to get the gross overall view of an object or upcoming word in a sentence. It is then sampled again to extract detailed information from the object or word. The two systems originate in the retinal ganglion cells (Solan, 1994). The system that is involved in the detailed analysis is called the *sustained system* (P cells) and is also called the *parvocellular system*. This is active during the fixation. The sustained system's role is an identification of shape, patterns and the resolution of fine detail. P cells comprise 80% of the retinal ganglion cells and are concentrated at the fovea. They have small receptive fields and are more responsive to low temporal (slow movement) and high spatial frequency (close together or detailed information) (Solan, 1994). Visual acuity and color vision are principally sustained system's functions (Garzia, 1990).

The visual system that operates with the sustained system is called the *transient system* (M cells). It is also called the *magnocellular system*. M cells comprise 10% of the retinal ganglion cells, are distributed evenly across the retina (Solan, 1994), and have large receptive fields (Bassi, 1990). The transient system is thought to be involved in the perception of motion, depth, brightness discrimina-

tion, the control of eye movements, and the localization of targets in space. It seems to function to accomplish a quick global analysis of a visual scene. It performs a global analysis of the incoming stimulus, breaking the field into units and regions and coding the position and movement of objects in space (Williams, 1990). Two of the primary functions of the transient system is that it carries motion detection and ocular motor control information (Garzia, 1990).

The role of the transient system in reading is critical. Previously, I have mentioned that the sustained system during the fixation is processing detailed information about the text. It is during the fixation that word encoding and decoding occur. The words are identified and the visual information is used for comprehension. When we pause to fixate during reading, both visual and cognitive information is used. Cognitive information is held in our subconscious to help in word identification and comprehension. When we move our eyes from one fixation to another by saccadic eye movement, the cognitive information continues; however, the visual information is terminated. If it isn't terminated at the end of the fixation, you will have visual information from one fixation smearing into the next fixation like an after image, making the text appear superimposed or overlapping (Lovegrove, 1990) (Figure 3-4). This is called *visible persistence* and can greatly interfere with reading. The reason why this does not happen is that the stimulation of the transient system generated by the start of the saccade inhibits (suppresses) the visible persistence of the sustained system from the pervious fixation (Solan, 1998). A deficit that affects the timing of either system will interfere with the processing of the second fixation and could lead to superimposition of successive inputs (Solan, 1994). This is what often happens with children with reading disabilities. In fact, over 75% of children with a reading disability manifest a transient defect (Lovegrove, 1990). Since inputs from successive fixations would be superimposed, disabled readers would do better in reading that does not require eye movements.

Transient deficits can cause the following problems:

1. Readers may only see parts of words.

2. If they do not know which fixation the information came from, they would know very little about the spatial arrangement of the letters and this could lead to reading errors and word or letter reversals.

3. It would be very difficult to learn any systematic grapheme to phoneme (phonics) rule if the appearance of the graphemes was in some way unstable.

4. The disabled reader may make repeated errors in different readings of the same word (Lovegrove, 1990).

5. The disabled reader may experience perceptual grouping deficits.

6. Readers may suffer an inability to selectively attend.

7. Readers may require larger time intervals to make accurate temporal judgments.

8. They may require more time to alleviate attention across visual space without eye movements.

9. Readers may skip lines during reading.

10. Readers may have to use a finger to help keep place during reading.

11. They may complain of words appearing to move on the page (Garzia, 1993).

It is important that we understand the relationship between the sustained and transient systems. It gives us a much better understanding as to why we do certain activities. This will become clearer when you follow the pathways of the two systems in the brain. For this description, I will use P cells to describe the sustained system and M cells to describe the transient system. These two parallel processing pathways in the visual system are relatively independent. These pathways transmit information from the retina to the dorsal lateral geniculate nucleus to the visual cortex and then to higher cortical levels with little or no cross-talk between them (Steinman, 1996). Although the principle function of the lateral geniculate nucleus is to relay ganglion cell information to the visual cortex, less than 20% of the synaptic input to the lateral geniculate nucleus is retinal in origin. The majority of the afferent neurons is extraretinal, midbrain, and brain stem; therefore, M and P ganglion cell information is influenced by nonvisual inputs (Solan, 1994). This is another reason why we do a lot of nonvisual activities that involve lower brain areas, such as motor activities.

Information travels faster along large, highly myelinated axons, causing information from the M pathway to reach the visual cortex faster than information from the P pathway (Steinman, 1996). Receiving information first from the M system and then from the P system allows the visual system first to quickly locate objects and then identify them (Steinman, 1996).

It seems obvious from the previous discussions that the proper functioning of the transient system is critical for normal reading skills. It also seems obvious that anything that can improve the transient system would be beneficial. Research has shown that the transient system is sensitive to short wavelengths (e. g., blue) (Solan, 1994) and may perform more efficiently when stimulated by this wavelength. One research paper showed that blue overlays significantly improved reading comprehension in 70% of children identified as reading disabled (Solan, 1998). Positive results were obtained by gray overlays but

they were not as successful as the blue overlays (Solan, 1998). It has also been shown that while blue enhances transient function, red reduces it (Richman, 1992). Does this mean that the Scotopic Sensitivity Syndrome exists? Also called the Irlen Syndrome, this claims that some children have difficulty processing full-spectrum light efficiency and that certain colored tints may improve their reading efficiency. This syndrome consists of eyestrain, photophobia (preference to reading in dim light), problems in visual resolution (blurred print, unstable text), restricted span of focus (only small areas of print seen), difficulties with sustained focusing (print blurs unless the reader puts a lot of effort into keeping it clear), problems in depth perception (difficulty judging distances), and handwriting (Garzia, 1990). The problem is there is no scientific evidence of a Scotopic Sensitivity Syndrome. All of the symptoms of this syndrome listed above are usually caused by visual problems such as ocular motor, convergence, or accommodation. What is important to know is that there does seem to be improvement in some children with a blue tint, but not necessarily other tints.

This chapter was devoted to eye movements and reading. It is extremely important that you have an understanding of eye movements and reading and also the sustained and transient systems. This enables you to understand how some visual procedures improve a child's overall reading efficiency.

Tips for a Successful Activities Program

There are no exercises that have been proven to enhance the transient system. Because of this, I recommend that we do exercises that affect the functions of the transient system and hope by doing this that the transient system is improved. Therefore, I recommend the following:

1. Do activities that work with the peripheral visual system.

2. Do a lot of visual scanning activities.

3. Do figure-ground activities; for example, hidden pictures, etc.

4. Try a light blue filter and see if this helps the child's reading performance. This can be obtained from an office supply store, usually as a page separator or file cover.

5. Do a lot of ocular motor activities.

References

Bassi, C. J. (1990). Clinical implications of parallel visual pathways. *Journal of the American Optometric Association, 61*(2), 98-109.

Ciuffreda, K. J. (1995). *Eye movement basics for the clinician*. New York: C.V. Mosby.

Edelman, G. M. (1998). Building a picture of the brain. *Daedalas, 127*(2), 37-69.

Evans, B. J. W. (1990). Review of ophthalmic factors in dyslexia. *Ophthal Physiol Opt, 10*, 123-132.

Fischer, B. (1993). Saccadic eye movements of dyslexic adult subjects. *Neuropsychologia, 31*(9), 887-906.

Garzia, R. P. (1994). Vision and reading II: Eye movements. *Journal of Optometric Vision Development, 25*, 4-26.

Garzia, R. P. (1993). Vision and reading I: Neuroanatomy and electrophysiology. *Journal of Vision Development, 24*, 4-51.

Garzia, R. P. (1990). Visual function and reading disability: An optometric viewpoint. *Journal of the American Optometric Association, 61*(2), 88-97.

Hoffman, J. E. (1995). The role of attention in saccadic eye movements. *Perception and Psychophysics, 5*, 787-795.

Krueger, L. E. (1993). Detection of letter repetition in words and nonwords: The effect of prior knowledge of repetition location. *American Journal of Psychology, 106*(1), 81.

Lovegrove, W. J. (1990). Experimental evidence for a transient system deficit in specific reading disability. *Journal of the Optometric Association, 61*(2), 137-146.

Moore, T. (1999). Shape representations and visual guidance of saccadic eye movements. *Science, 285*, 5435.

Morris, H. F. (1973). *Manual for the edl/biometrics reading eye II*. New York: McGraw-Hill, Inc.

Rayner, K. (1983). *Eye movements in reading*. New York: Academic Press.

Richman, J. (1992). Annual review of the literature 1991. *Journal of Optometric Vision Development, 23*, 3-37.

Smith, F. (1994). *Understanding reading*. Mahwah, NJ: Lawrence Erlbaum Associates.

Solan, H. A. (2001). Role of visual attention in cognitive control of oculomotor readiness in students with reading disabilities. *Journal of Learning Disabilities, 34*(2), 107.

Solan, H. A. (1998). Eye movement efficiency in normal and reading disabled elementary school children: Effects of varying luminance and wavelength. *Journal of the American Optometric Association, 69*(7), 455-464.

Solan, H. A. (1994). Transient and sustained processing. *Journal of Behavioral Optometry, 5*(6), 149-154.

Stanovich, K. E. (1993). Understanding and teaching reading: An interactive model. *American Journal of Psychology, 106*(3), 456.

Steinman, B. A. (1996). Vision and reading III: Visual attention. *Journal of Optometric Vision Development, 27*, 4-28.

Vogel, G. L. (1995). Saccadic eye movements: Theory testing and therapy. *Journal of Behavioral Optometry, 6*(1), 3-12.

Williams, M. C. (1990). Perceptual consequences of a temporal processing deficit in reading disabled children. *Journal of the American Optometric Association, 61*(2), 111-121.

Ygge, J. (1994). *Eye movements in reading*. Oxford, England: Elsevier Science, Inc.

Chapter Four

OCULAR MOTOR

The function of eye movements goes well beyond vision and reflects higher brain processes. (Gauthier, 1990)

One of the most important areas of a successful activities program is ocular motor. It is one of the easiest areas of the visual system to train and it has the greatest impact on school performance, especially in reading. Ocular motor consists of control and coordination of eye movements. Deficits can severely impair a child's ability to effectively scan his environment, and in turn, devastate him functionally (Wolff, 1973). Ocular motor dysfunction is one of the main causes of inefficient reading and can directly affect reading speed. In my opinion, no other area can have as drastic an effect on school performance, and as a result have as positive an effect on school performance when it is remediated.

Eye movements are the fastest and most frequent movements made by the human body. The eye movement control system is complex, sophisticated, and advanced. It is erroneous to solely equate eye movements with vision. The function of eye movements goes well beyond vision and reflects higher brain processes. In order to localize an object in space, the central nervous system (CNS) must use a combination of visual (retinal) information and a knowledge of the position of the eye in its orbit. Part of this is based on sensing the motor commands to the ocular muscles and part on sensing proprioceptive inputs from the ocular muscles themselves. For large ocular deviations, ocular muscle proprioception may account for 32% of the information used to sense eye position (Gauthier, Year).

The ocular motor system directs both eyes toward the object to be viewed. Eye movements are controlled by three pairs of muscles, the medial and lateral recti, inferior and superior obliques, and inferior and superior recti. Medial and lateral recti of each eye contract reciprocally to move the eyes from side to side. The superior and inferior recti move the eyes up and down. The obliques are responsible for rotating the eyeballs to keep the visual image upright. The ocular motor system places and holds the eyes on target by six classes of movements: fixations, vestibular, optokinetic, smooth pursuit, saccades, and vergence.

1. *Fixations*: holds the image of a stationary object on the fovea.
2. *Vestibulo-ocular reflex*: holds images of the seen world steady on the retina during brief head rotations.
3. *Optokinetic*: holds images of the seen world steady on the retina during sustained and low frequency head rotations gaze shifting.
4. *Smooth pursuit*: holds the image of a moving target on the fovea.
5. *Saccades*: directs images of eccentrically located objects of interest onto the fovea.
6. *Vergence*: moves the eyes in opposite directions so that images of a single object are placed simultaneously on the foveas and the images of both eyes "fuse" into one image.

Oculomotor stress symptoms include intermittent blurred vision, diplopia, visual fatigue, orbital aching, eye burning, and headaches. The visual subjective symptoms include:

1. Intermittent and/or sustained blurred vision.
2. Intermittent and/or sustained diplopia, trembling visual images, problems in following, and/or shifting lines during reading.
3. Eyes burning, tearing, orbital pain, visual fatigue, headaches, aching neck/shoulders, and/or nausea (Oslo, 1989).

When we work with children, we are mainly concerned with three ocular motor areas. These are smooth pursuit, saccades, and vergence. It is important that we remember that the sole purpose of the ocular motor system is to keep the image that we are looking at on both foveas at the same time. If this doesn't happen, then we get the symptoms mentioned above. At this point, before we continue, I think that we need to have a good understanding of the anatomy of the eye, especially the foveal area.

Light enters our eye through the cornea, which is the main refractory part of the eye. An irregularly shaped cornea is the main cause of astigmatism. After the cornea, the light passes through the pupil and through the lens. The lens of the eye is a transparent biconvex body of crystalline appearance (crystal clear). The color of the lens changes with age. In the infant and young adult, it is quite colorless. After about 35 years, the central portion gets a definite yellow tinge, which becomes darker and more extensive as time goes on. In the older person, the lens often has an amber color (Wolff, 1973). If there is an opacity in the lens, this is called a *cataract*. The diameter of the lens is 9 to 10 mm, and its thickness (from 4 to 5 mm) varies greatly as the eye is focused for distant or near objects (accommodation) (Zoltan, 1996). Light then passes through the vitreous humour. This is a transparent, colorless, gelatinous mass of a consistency somewhat firmer than egg white which fills the posterior four-fifths of the globe (Wolff, 1973). The light then hits the *retina*, which is the posterior portion of the eye (Figures 4-1 and 4-2). The image that hits the retina should be a sharp image. It is the responsibility of the anterior position of the eye to make the image as sharp as possible (the cornea and lens). This image is the adequate stimulus that excites the sensory receptors of the retina. The differences in light intensity of the image produce different levels of pigment breakdown to which the photoreceptors respond

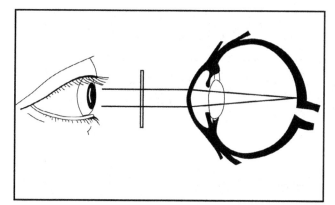

Figure 4-1. The pathway of light as it enters the eye and focuses on the fovea.

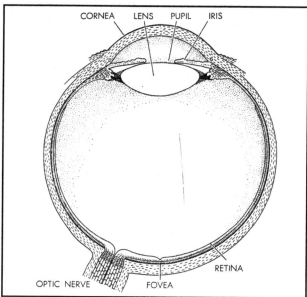

Figure 4-2. The fovea is only 1.5 mm in diameter. Reprinted with permission of Eric Mose, Jr.

correspondingly. They transform the energy of the stimulus into nerve impulses that are conducted by the optic nerve fibers to appropriate cell stations in the brain. The visual receptors in the retina are the rods and cones (Moses, 1970).

The rods get their name from their outer segment, which is rod-like. The cones derive their name from their shape, which resembles a flask with a narrow neck. There are about 120 million rods in the retina and 6 million cones. In man and higher mammals, the central region of the retina or macula differs considerably from the surrounding retina. The center of the macula (the fovea) contains only cones and no rods. The number of cones decreases rapidly from the center, falling to a low value in the periphery. While the number of cones decreases the further from the fovea you go, the number of rods increases. The rods respond to light of low intensity and for the registration of movement in the periphery, while the cones are used for color vision and discrimination of fine detail (Wolff, 1973). In order for a person to discriminate fine detail, the light that enters the eye must focus on the fovea. The fovea is 1.5 mm in diameter (Shapero, 1968).

When we read, the visual image must fall on the fovea for letter identification to occur. If it does not fall directly on the fovea, there are fewer cones to help identify the letter. For example, if we are directly fixating on a letter, that letter is being sampled by something like a grid of 30 x 30 cones (also called feature detectors), two letters further out in our peripheral vision, a letter is being sampled by a 19 x 19 grid of feature detectors two letters further out by a grid of 15 x 15 feature detectors. Because the brain does not have enough feature detectors, we cannot identify letters more than 4 to 6 positions from the point of fixation. Letters will compete for available feature detectors. This is called "crowding" (Elsendoorn, 1979). As wonderful as the human brain is, it can't handle all the visual images to which it is exposed. It must be selective and make full use of the feature detectors that it has available. In fact, three-quarters of the visual information

available to the brain when we read is ignored (Smith, 1994). Because the brain can't handle all the visual information that is available, it sends the eyes to the point of the object or word that gives it the most information. It has to maximize its available time and the limited number of feature detectors. For example, we know that the tops of letters and the beginning of words supply the most useful information (Pirozzolo, 1981). This is why the eye usually fixates on a letter near the front of a word. Because of the limited amount of feature detectors, the eye is constantly in motion (Figure 4-3). It never stays still. Small, involuntary movements persist even when the eye is "fixed" on a stationary object. As a result, the image of the object on the retina is kept in constant motion. One movement the eye makes is a slow drift away from the center of the fovea. The drifting motion terminates in a flick that brings the image back toward the center of the fovea. Superimposed on the drift motion is a tremor with frequencies up to 150 cycles per second and amplitude of about half a cone receptor (Pritchard, 1961). To prove that the eye spends more time on the areas of objects or letters that give it the most information, an experiment was conducted in the 1950s that stabilized the movements of the eye. What the experiment found was that when the eye did not move, the image the eye was looking at slowly faded away. However, the area of the image or word that faded away last was the area that gave the most information. In other words, the eye spends more time on the areas that supply it the most information because it has a limited amount of feature detectors.

When we see an object, the brain lays down scan paths. These are memory traces that the brain will need to

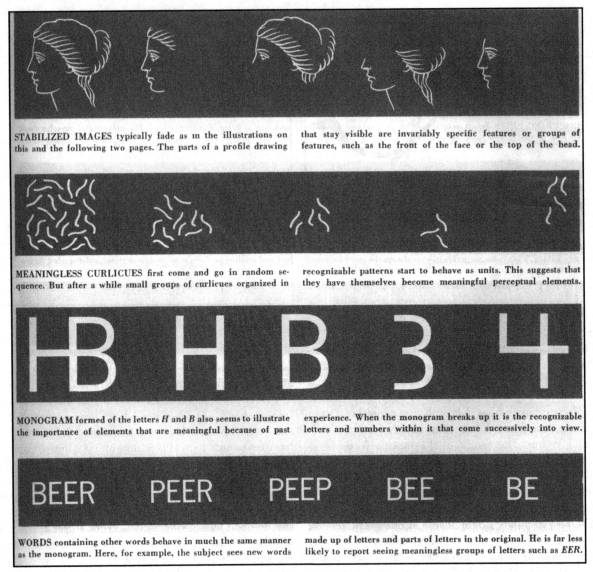

STABILIZED IMAGES typically fade as in the illustrations on this and the following two pages. The parts of a profile drawing that stay visible are invariably specific features or groups of features, such as the front of the face or the top of the head.

MEANINGLESS CURLICUES first come and go in random sequence. But after a while small groups of curlicues organized in recognizable patterns start to behave as units. This suggests that they have themselves become meaningful perceptual elements.

MONOGRAM formed of the letters *H* and *B* also seems to illustrate the importance of elements that are meaningful because of past experience. When the monogram breaks up it is the recognizable letters and numbers within it that come successively into view.

WORDS containing other words behave in much the same manner as the monogram. Here, for example, the subject sees new words made up of letters and parts of letters in the original. He is far less likely to report seeing meaningless groups of letters such as *EER*.

Figure 4-3. The eye spends more time on the areas of an object that give it the most information, as you can see on the bottom image of the word BEER. The last areas that fade out are the first two letters, as we know the first letters in a word supply the most information to help identify the word. The last areas that fade out with letters are the angles that form the letters. Reprinted with permission from Eric Mose, Jr.

help identify the object the next time it sees it. The way you scan an object may be different from the way I scan an object but what is important is that scan paths are put into our memory. You don't have to physically move your eye to generate scan paths. There is also internal scanning, as for example, when you look at a printed letter. When we see the object or letter the next time, we will scan it the same way. This is why activities that emphasize proper visual scanning of letters or words are extremely important.

There are three conclusions that can be made about the recognition of objects. First, the internal representation or memory of an object is a piecemeal affair: an assemblage of features or more strictly of memory traces of features. Second, the features of an object are the parts of it (such as angles and curves of line drawings) that yield the most information. Third, the memory traces recording the features are assembled into the complete internal representation being connected by other memory traces that record the shifts of attention required to pass from feature to feature, either by eye movements or with internal shifts of attention (Noton, 1971).

The extraocular muscles have only one function, and that is to fixate the visual image on the fovea. They must move in a coordinated manner to get the visual image on both foveas at the exact same time. If the light from both eyes does not get to both foveas at the same time, the child will experience blurred or double vision. For the child to be successful in school, efficient visual skills must be obtained. The three ocular motor areas that we work with are smooth pursuit, saccadic fixations, and vergence. This book will include activities for smooth pursuit and saccadic fixations.

Smooth pursuit eye movements enable continuous clear vision of moving objects. This visual following reflex produces eye movements that assure continuous foveal fixation of objects moving in space. The maximum pursuit velocities are approximately 60 degrees per second. Pursuit eye movements are only involved when a target is moving (Scheiman, 1994). Pursuit movements allow primates to use visual inputs related to image motion (defined as target motion with respect to the eye) and to drive smooth eye movement that keeps the eyes pointed at small moving targets (Krauzlis, 1991). If a child is sitting in a chair and following a swinging ball on a string or if he is playing baseball and following the flight of the ball before he catches it, these actions constitute smooth pursuit eye movements. The pursuit system is clearly functional by 7 weeks of age (Bennett, 1996), but is not fully developed until the age of 16 to 18 (Snashall, 1983). Three different visual signals provide the commands for smooth eye acceleration. These signals are related to image velocity, the abrupt onset of image motion, and changes in image velocity (Krauzlis, 1991). Although pursuit movements are not used in reading, there have been investigations of their integrity in the reading disabled. If pursuit deficits are found, it suggests that a generalized oculomotor deficit may exist in disabled readers (Garzia, 1994). Smooth pursuit abnormalities are significantly more prevalent in dyslexia (Grinberg, 1978). Only 8% of normal subjects have abnormal smooth pursuit movements (Levin, 1982); however, the number is much higher with dyslexic children. Eye movements of children identified as dyslexic are much more erratic than those of normal children. These findings are indicative of a malfunctioning ocular motor control system or a more general problem in sequencing (Punnett, 1984). Symptoms of poor pursuits are excessive head movement during reading and poor performance in sports (Scheiman, 1994). Symptoms when you are observing a child include jerking eye movements or midline tremors as the eye crosses its midline. Smooth pursuit eye movements are easy to test but require some practice. To test a child, have him seated in front of you at a distance of a little over arm's length. Test monocularly (one eye at a time) by covering one of his eyes. Hold a fixation object, such as a pencil, directly in front of the child and slowly move it in a horizontal direction going left to right and then right to left. Have

the child follow it with his eye and remind him not to move his body or his head. Go out to his periphery and make the left to right movements at least 2 feet in length. Have him wear his glasses if he needs them but make sure you don't go too far in his periphery that he loses the target because of the edge of his eyeglass frame. You need to look for any excessive losses in fixation or large midline tremors. Also make a note if you feel the child is losing the target due to poor concentration. Repeat the same procedures with his other eye. Make a note if you feel one eye is worse. You can also do it binocularly to see if there are any restrictions in eye movement; however, pursuit testing for poor ocular motor is done monocularly.

The second ocular motor movement that we are going to discuss is saccadic fixation. Remember that smooth pursuit refers to smooth tracking eye movements that permit continuous foveation of objects that are moving in space (Leigh, 1983). Saccadic fixations are rapid eye movements to stationary objects, such as moving our eyes across a page when we read. Saccades are eye movements that enable us to rapidly redirect our line of sight so that the point of interest stimulates the fovea. Saccade is a French word for "jerk" (Smith, 1994). They are the fastest eye movements with velocities as high as 700 degrees per second (1/25 to 1/50 of a second) (Griffin, 1974). Saccades may be inaccurate in two ways. The most common inaccuracy is a slight undershot, and a less common inaccuracy is overshot (Scheiman, 1994). However, they are normally accurate within a few tenths of a degree under normal conditions (Collewijn, 1988). The brain programs saccadic eye movements as a pulse-step process. The pulse is a velocity command that overcomes the vicious drag on the eye due to its surrounding orbital tissues. The step command is a position command that holds the eye in the correct position against the elasticity of the orbital tissues, which tend to pull the eye back to the central position. It has been shown that the stiffness in the left eye when it is rotated in the nasal direction is about 11% greater than if it is rotated in the temporal direction (Collewijn, 1988). The brain must continuously monitor eye position so that appropriate commands for saccades can be made. To do this, the brain monitors both visual inputs and eye position. It appears that the cerebellum calibrates both the amplitude of the saccade as well as the pulse step. The command then has information not only about the speed but also about the direction and final position and thus the saccade is accurate (Downey, Year).

The process of saccades is very complicated when you consider that both eyes must be coordinated to arrive at their targets at the exact same time. Binocular saccades have been shown to have an abduction–adduction asymmetry. *Abduction* means away from midline or temporally, while *adduction* is toward midline or nasally. It has been shown that the saccades of the abducting eye consistently had a larger size, a higher velocity, a shorter duration, and were more skewed than the adducting saccades of the fellow eye. As a result, the eyes diverge by as much as 3 degrees during horizontal saccades. It has also been noted that there appears to be postsaccadic drift so that the fovea of each eye is guided towards the target (Collewijn, 1988). The purpose of this drift is to correctly put the image of both eyes on their foveas.

When we move our eyes from point to point in space, there is no visual perception during these movements. This was first noticed in 1898 (Martin, 1974). In other words, there is no blurred visual image during the saccade. The threshold for detecting visual information is raised during the saccadic movement. Our visual acuity decreases to 20/1000 (Ciuffreda, 1995) so that no visual image is noticed. This is called saccadic suppression and starts at 20 msec prior to and 75 msec after the onset of the saccade (Rayner, 1983). If this was not done, we would notice blurred visual images as our eyes moved. The cause of the saccadic suppression is the retinal stimulation generated by the movement of the eye (Martin, 1974). This is easy to confirm. Stand in front of a mirror and quickly move your eyes back and forth. You will not see your eyes move.

Saccadic eye movement appears to develop during 2 to 5 months of age (Matsuzawa, 2001). It has been observed that children younger than 7 years often have inadequate eye movements. Most 5 year olds have difficulty performing accurate saccadic eye movements. Most children show marked improvement until 7. After that age, improvement slows down considerably. These findings suggest that maturation of the parts of the brain responsible for sequential control of saccadic sequential systems may constitute a prerequisite for the accurate execution of sequential tasks such as reading (Pavlidis, 1985).

Many symptoms of saccadic dysfunction are associated with reading. These include head movements, frequent loss of place, omission of words, skipping lines, slow reading speed, and poor comprehension. Children who have these symptoms also have difficulty copying from the chalkboard and have difficulty solving math problems with columns of numbers (Scheiman, 1994). Most dyslexic children have these symptoms and you will find most of them have very poor saccadic fixations. By improving children's eye movements, you can be very successful in improving children's reading speed and efficiency and improving their quality of life by making school and especially reading easier for them.

Tips for a Successful Ocular Motor Therapy Program

1. Start with smooth pursuit training.
2. Always start monocular. When you feel each eye is performing on the same level, proceed to binocular.
3. Make sure there is no head or body movement by the child. If he moves his head or body, make a note of this, as it shows immaturity in separating gross and fine motor skills.
4. Start saccadic fixation training in open space. For example, saccadic fixation between hand held pencils. When you feel the child can do these fairly well, proceed to "on paper" saccadic fixation, such as tracking across a page of print.

References

Bennett, B. (1996). Origins and early development of perception, action and representation. *Annual Review of Psychology*, 47, 431(29).

Ciuffreda, K. J. (1995). *Eye movement basics for the clinician*. New York: C.V. Mosby.

Collewijn, H. (1988). Binocular co-ordination of human horizontal saccadic eye movements. *Journal of Physiology, 404*, 157-182.

Downey, D. L. Eye movements: Pathophysiology, examination and clinical importance. *Journal of Neuroscience Nursing*, 30(1), 15(10).

Elsendoorn, G. (1979). *Toward the use of eye movements in the study of language processing*. Technical Report No. 134, COVD Paper, No. 174968.

Garzia, R. P. (1994). Vision and reading II. *Journal of Optometric Vision Development, 25*, 4-26.

Gauthier, G. M. (1990). The role of ocular muscle proprioception in visual localization of targets. *Science*, 249(4964), 58(4).

Griffin, D. C. (1974). Saccades as related to reading disorders. *Journal of Learning Disabilities*, 7(5).

Grinberg, D. A. (1978). Eye movements, scan paths and dyslexia. *American Journal of Optometry*, 55(8), 557-570.

Krauzlis, R. J. (1991). Visual motion commands for pursuit eye movements in the cerebellum. *Science*, 253(5019), 568.

Leigh, J. R. (1983). *The neurology of eye movement*. Philadelphia: F. A. Davis Company.

Levin, S. (1982). Identification of abnormal patterns in eye movements of schizophrenic patients. *Archives of General Psychiatry, 39*, 1125-1130.

Martin, E. (1974). Saccadic suppression. *Psychological Bulletin*, 81(12), 899-917.

Matsuzawa, M. (2001). Development of saccade target selection in infants. *Perceptual and Motor Skills, 93,* 115-123.

Moses, R. A. (1970). *Adler's physiology of the eye.* St. Louis, MO: C.V. Mosby Co.

Noton, D. (1971). Eye movements and visual perception. Scientific American, Perception: Mechanisms and Models; 219-227.

Oslo, I. L. (1989). Visual anomalies, visually related problems and reading difficulty. *Optometrie, 4.*

Pavlidis, G. T. (1985). Eye movement differences between dyslexics, normal, and retarded readers while sequentially fixating digits. *American Journal of Optometry and Physiological Optics, 62*(12), 820-832.

Pirozzolo, F. (1981). *Neuropsychological and cognitive processes in reading.* New York: Academic Press.

Pritchard, R. M. (1961). Stabilized images on the retina. Scientific America, Perception: Mechanisms and Models, 176-182.

Punnett, A. F. (1984). Relationship between reinforcement and eye movements during ocular motor training with learning disabled children. *Journal of Learning Disabilities, 17*(1), 16-19.

Rayner, K. (1983). *Eye movements in reading.* New York: Academic Press.

Scheiman, M. (1994). *Clinical management of binocular vision.* Philadelphia: J. B. Lippincott Co.

Shapero, M. (1968). *Dictionary of visual science.* Seattle, WA: Chilton Book Company.

Snashall, S. E. (1983). Vestibular function tests in children. *Journal of the Royal Society of Medicine, 76*(7), 555-559.

Smith, F. (1994). *Understanding reading.* Mahwah, NJ: Lawrence Erlbaum Associates.

Wolff, E. (1973). *Anatomy of the eye and orbit.* Philadelphia: W. B. Saunders Co.

Zoltan, B. (1996). *Vision, perception, and cognition.* Thorofare, NJ: SLACK Incorporated.

Form OM-1
COLORED OVERLAYS

Purpose: Stimulation of the transient system.

Materials: Light blue plastic. These can often be found as page dividers in office supply stores.

Method: Have the child do the activity below.

Levels 2 to 5: Lay the plastic overlay over the child's reading material. Ask him if he feels this helps him and makes reading easier. If it does, have him continue to use this with his reading assignments. If it does not, do not use it.

Form OM-2
FIGURE GROUND

Purpose: Stimulation of the transient system.

Materials: Hidden picture magazines and games like *Where's Waldo?*; also, *Highlights* magazine offers a lot of hidden pictures activities.

Method: Have the child do the activities below.

Levels 1 to 2: Use the *Highlights* magazines or *Where's Waldo?* books.

Levels 3 to 5: Use normal reading material. Designate a letter (for example, R) and ask the child to look at the page of print and circle as many R's as he can. Vary the letters he is to find. Time him and see how fast he can find the designated letter. You can vary this and ask him to find blends or circle all the words with "tion" in them or that end with "ing".

Form OM-3
STATIC FIXATION

Purpose: Visual attention.

Materials: None.

Method: Have the child do the following activities to improve his fixation skills.

Levels 1 to 3:
1. Have the child lie on his back with his head up. Mark a spot high on the wall for him to look at. Stand over the child and pull him to a sitting position. The child should never take his eyes off the spot on the wall.
2. Have the child sit and rock back and forth without taking his eyes off the spot on the wall.
3. As the child is standing, have him walk around and not take his eyes off the spot on the wall.
4. As the child is standing and looking at the spot on the wall, have him jump completely around and pick up a spot on the opposite wall.

Form OM-4
LINE COUNTING

Purpose: Ocular motor.

Materials: Paper, pencil.

Method: Draw a series of lines on a sheet of paper. You may want to start with the lines spread out until the child becomes good at this activity.

Levels 1 to 2:
1. Ask the child to touch each line and count them in a left to right sequence. See how fast he can count the correct number of lines.
2. Have the child count the lines without touching the paper with his pencil. See how fast he can count the correct number of lines.

Form OM-5
FIXATION ACTIVITIES

Purpose: Ocular motor.

Materials: Marker board, metronome.

Method: For these activities, the child is only to move his eyes. There should not be any head or body movement. Do these activities at first one eye at a time (cover his other eye). When he can do the activities without difficulty one eye at a time, have him do both eyes together.

Level 1:
1. Have the child sit with his arms extended in front of him and thumbs up. At your command, he is to shift his eyes accurately and quickly from one thumb to the other. Have him continue going back and forth between thumbs. Make sure he does not move his head or body.
2. Have the child seated at a table with his hands folded in front of him, thumbs up. The child looks at an object to the left of his thumb, then his left thumb, right thumb, and an object to the right of his right thumb. Always go in a left to right direction.
3. Draw two Xs on the blackboard at eye level about 3 feet apart. Have the child stand centered between the two Xs and about 2 feet in front of the board. At the beat of the metronome, have him quickly move his eyes back and forth from one X to the other.

Levels 2 to 3:
1. Have the child seated at a table. At the beat of the metronome, he is to look quickly from an object on the wall to the left of the table, to an object on the table, to an object on the wall to the right of the table. The table should be about 15 to 20 feet from the wall. Vary the number of objects. Make sure he moves his eyes only, not his head or body.

Form OM-6
FOUR CORNER FIXATION

Purpose: Ocular motor.

Materials: Marker board, metronome.

Method: The child will stand approximately 5 feet from an X drawn on the marker board at eye level. Set the metronome at about 60 beats a minute. He is to move his eyes only, not his head or body.

Level 1: Without the metronome, point to the corners where you want him to look. For example, when you point to the top right corner, he will move his eyes quickly and accurately to the right corner. He then moves his eyes back to the X and waits for your next instruction.

Levels 2 to 3:
1. The child will look at the X target for four beats, then on a corner of the marker board for four beats, then to the X for four beats, then the next corner for four beats. This is done until he has looked at all four corners. Start with the top right and work to bottom right, bottom left, and top left.
2. Have him repeat #1, but he is to call out the direction of the corners as he looks at them. For example, "top right", "bottom right", etc.

Levels 4 to 5: Set the metronome to about 30 beats a minute. At the first beat, he calls out the direction he is to move his eyes. For example, top right and looks at that corner, points to the corner on the second beat, puts his arm down on the third beat and looks at the center X on the fourth beat.

Form OM-7
PENCIL PURSUITS

Purpose: Ocular motor.

Materials: Pencil, finger puppet.

Method: Start by doing the activity one eye at a time (cover one of the child's eyes) and then both eyes at the same time. For younger children use a finger puppet, and for older children use a pencil. Have the child seated about 36 inches in front of you. Slowly move your pencil. He is to follow it with his eyes only. The child is not to move his head or body. Don't use both eyes until he can do each eye individually without any difficulty.

Level 1: Have the child follow your pencil with his eyes. You can go left to right, vertically or diagonally. The following are the different patterns you can use.

Level 2: Have the child follow your pencil with his eyes. Do the same activities as Level 1, but also move your pencil in circular patterns, e. g., circles or lazy eights.

Levels 3 to 5: Same as Level 2, but as the child is doing the activities, ask him questions about his peripheral vision. For example: "As you are following the pencil, without taking your eyes off the pencil, how many chairs are at the table"?

Form OM-8
NUMBER PURSUITS

Purpose: Ocular motor.

Materials: Metronome, large index cards with up to 12 numbers printed on them.

Method: Start by having the child do this activity with one eye at a time (cover his other eye). After he can do this activity easily with one eye, have him use both eyes at the same time. Have him call out the digits in a left to right sequence. He is not to move his head or body, only his eyes. Hold the card about 3 feet from the child.

Level 2:
1. Have him call out the digits in a left to right sequence.
2. As he is calling out the digits, move the card slowly in a circular motion.

Level 3:
1. Have him call out the digits in a left to right sequence. Set the metronome to about 60 beats per minute. Each time he hears a beat, he calls out a digit.
2. Same as # 1, but move the card slowly in a circular motion.

Form OM-9
GLOBAL SCANNING

Purpose: To train the transient system.

Materials: Make a group of flash cards with the following type of patterns on them. Think up as many variations as you can.

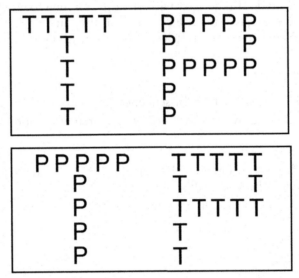

Levels 1 and 2: Use the cards in group "a". Flash the card at the child (a flash is 2 seconds), and ask him to tell you the identification of the big letter. Also, sometimes ask him to identify one of the little letters.

Levels 3 and 4: Use the shapes in group "b". Ask him to tell you the identification of the large letter. Remember to flash the card, don't let him see it for more than 2 seconds. For example:

```
        P P P P P
            P
            P
            P
            P
```

would be identified as a "T". Vary this by asking him to identify one of the small letters.

Level 5:
1. Use the following type shapes:

```
    d                       b
    d                       b
    d                       b
    d d d d         b b b b
```

The instructions are the same as Levels 3 to 4.

Form OM-10
LETTER SEARCH

Purpose: To train global processing.

Materials: Normal reading material.

Method: Have the child do the following activity.

Levels 2 to 5:
The child is to circle all words where a letter appears twice. This can be varied by finding words with three letters or words where there are no letters that appear more than once. For younger children, use larger print books. The child is to scan in a left to right direction on each line of print. He is not to randomly search or use his finger as a marker to keep his place.

Form OM-11
WORDS IN WORDS

Purpose: To train the transient system by global to fine visual processing.

Materials: Reading materials.

Method: Have the child do the following activity.

Levels 3 to 5: Have the child find as many words as he can that are hidden in other words. For example: many = man; other = the.

Form OM-12
Visual Scanning

Purpose: To train the transient system.

Materials: Use the pages given in this book.

Method: In each level, the child is to find and circle the letters or groups of letters given at the bottom of the page. He must locate and circle the letters in the same sequence as they are given at the bottom of the page. Keep a record of his time at the bottom of the page. Levels 1 to 3 are the whole page activities. Levels 4 to 5 are the half page activities; however, everyone should start with the first activity. In order for you to use these sheets more than once, put a clear plastic sheet over the page.

6   36   28

        12

                        49   45   27   47

35

40   7   9   37   29   46

                                    30

11   43   20

26 50

4   8   16   19   25

15

                  39

                        41   32   21

                  10

            1

18

                  24

            48   34   38   3

14   23

                        33

42

5 13

Find: 6, 7, 8, 9, 10   Min. _____ Sec. _____

Form OM-12 (continued)
Visual Scanning

6   36   28   12

49 45

27   35   7

40

          9

                              37

                    29

          46

                                                  30

11   43

                                                            50

20 26
4

                         19

8

          16

     25

39 41

10

                              21

     32

          1

24 48
18 34

38   14
3

          23

42 5
33

13
                         17

Find 36, 37, 38, 39, 40.   Min. _____ Sec. _____

Form OM-12 (continued)
VISUAL SCANNING

1   85   51   100   55   18
83 64
19
21
   94   36   30   46
     25   63   95   54

2 88   80

4   84
75   89   52   90   48
91
47   74   81
     73
20   37
     35   99
     53
37   94
     96   86   3   59   5
39   31
60   67   32   97
61   10
33   45   24   72   44
     68   62   11   65
   69   28   23
     76
43   70   16   66
   77
     34
   29   71   78   17
15   79   38   56
   12
     40   26   8   9
15   22   14   58   41   13   7

Find: 4, 77, 35, 2, 94, 37, 80, 31, 19, 62   Min. _____ Sec._____

Form OM-12 (continued)
VISUAL SCANNING

51   6   83   79   22
                    14   30   63
                        43   81   31
85
                        25   72   2
    41   62

99   64   82   66   48

    44   7   50   29   65
        21   80
    23   84   67   1

28   24   42   8
        98

    45   71   20   86   46

        26   100   73   69
87   3   47   97
                                27   19   61
                88
39   4   70   49   16   36

                                92   51   74
        93   18   89   96

                5   9   38
            52   17
91
            95   37   90   78
53   76   77
    54   35   94

34   10   11   58
32   59   60   13

Find: 32, 99, 71, 50, 1, 3, 6, 48, 9, 13   Min. _____ Sec. _____

Form OM-12 (continued)
VISUAL SCANNING

12   22   33   q   26   r   15   s
                 t   41   l   o   39   2
        46   n   32   21   30
        p   50   1   25   14 m
           3   49   40
               13   29
k   38
11   48   20   45
               a   u   v   b
                   23   47
        42   28   37
g   4   h   I   16   I   19
           31   5   6
        43   c   d   w   36
44
               7   8   24   9   35   10
17   34
               x   y   27   18   e   f   z

Find: 28, 38, 48, s, d, f, 14, 24, 34, 44   Min. ___ Sec. ___

        50   a   49   48   h
                   r   47   46   w
               45   44   b   43 42
41   j   n   40
                   q   u   39   v
               38   37   c   36   35
        34   33   x
32   s   m   31
        i   30   29   28   27   g
                   k   26   25
               d   24 23   22   o
p   21   20   19   f
18   t   17   y
        16   15   14 13   11
        10   9   8
7   6   5   4   3
2   e   I

Find: 33, 44, 22, 11, t, y, I, d, x, 10   Min. ____ Sec. ___

Form OM-12 (continued)
VISUAL SCANNING

z   34   3   29   19   w   g
  4   23   44   b
                         o   39
43   5   n   e
    18   f   42   6   m
  28   20 35   x   41
        11   r   a   30   7
        8 24   33   38
            40   10   17   21
q   27   c   v   1
  32   p   50
12   49 h 16   36   48 i
31   13   d   47   15
    u   46   q   25

14   t   j   22 45   y   2
         1   26   37   k

Find: a, 4, 7, w, 18, 29, e, t, 43, q   Min. _____   Sec. _____

---

    v   26   j 1 16   3   i   37
a   36   44   15   z   t
  2   35   25   u   6   h
20   50   b 24   k 14   43 y
  39   17 45   g   r   79
7   c   8   f
        38 27   d   4
  34   19   28   13   40   18
    s   l   42   w   48
    e   31   q 41   29
                          23   12
5   m 30   46   21   32   x
  9   n   10   33   47
o   p   11   22

Find: 17, h, 5, r, 31, 42, f, s, 6, o   Min. _____   Sec. ____

Form OM-12 (continued)
VISUAL SCANNING

cr   bl   wh   gq   sh

pl   uj sw   ls

cc   ll

al   cl   dr   tk

ni   we   ht   rt   eb

ed   rp xe

ba gn   mi ps   hc

rc   lb hw   hs lp   la

lc   gb   fv   rd

hy   zx

ex

nm   ab   io

ng   pp   im sp   ch

ng   hk

gh   yu   pw   in th

tr   be jj   de   qq

pr

Find: sp, cr, bl, th, ng   **Min. ___ Sec. ___**

---

qq

nt   ww   rm   sp

dw   ee   pa

st   yx   rr   ch

fo   tt   qa   yy   tc

uu

ii   cr   ji

wl   oo   in

aa   bl   ba ko wt bb

th

ff   dd   re nh   ll wh

gg

tx   rt   tr   js pp

sh   gy lf mm   mo

nn   he be

vv   pl   kp zz   ex de

pa   gj   dk   sl   al

wm   eo   pr

Find: ch, ex, be, sh, in   **Min. ____ Sec. ___**

Form OM-12 (continued)
VISUAL SCANNING

```
    fi           ha                    cl          ps      fr
te                      mi                                                    
        tw                  as        tr    bu                  lo
    cu                                cr    th
  we                          cp            be              nt      dr
        ge      .                     pt                    sm  sa
bl          al
        ir              in    ap            eq          qu      ch

                ou                          pa  fo  wh
        de              sp            is                        cd
le
                im          rt              pl
            so                  tc         ex              ph
ab                  sh  wp            ap
            ow                        de          pr      ne
os                      ci            ng          na
        fa                   ff                            me
            hi                              ev
        eb                        ct        ph
```

Find: **al, sp, be, tr, in**   **Min. ____ Sec. ____**

```
of           ap         fe        nu    tr          re          go
                          no    ga  mi
                                  tr          wh
        ch              cr                    bl
nu          di      sr        wr    su    te              br
                                              be
    im          ll  qu    sh          un              en
  am                      ho    pp            go
  rc          ng      wa              sc
xp            in      ai  av    xx    pl  su    bb  ny    ab      va
de    rr      dr          im        sp    st        ss
pr            th  xi                  al    ln        li              s y
re          ph    be        en              ct        ef
            ex                        cl
```

Find: **im, cr, ex, wh, bl**   **Min. ____ Sec. ____**

Form OM-12 (continued)
VISUAL SCANNING

```
qq                      pp
qp                      dd
                qp                      qd
                   bd                   dd
                 bp          bb
                   pp              bq
                      bb
qq                   dd              dp
       pp                                   dq

qd                      db        qb
              dd
bp                 pq              dd
                  pb                          pp
bq          pd                 dd
                      pp              pb
```

Find: bq, dp, pq, pd, qd   **Min.** ____ **Sec.** ___

```
pp                   qq              pp              bb
dd                qp
              dp
pq                   qb
       pp                      dq
                         bp
                   db          dp                   bd
              dd                          dd
                   qd
                 pq
           qb
pd          qq                pp
                   dd          dp                      pp
```

Find: pd, qd, dq, bb, pb   **Min.** ____ **Sec.** ____

Form OM-12 (continued)
VISUAL SCANNING

bd　　　　　　　bp　　　　dd　　　　　　　dq　　　　　　　　　bb

　　　　　　bq　　dd　　　　　　　bb　　　　pq
dp　　　　　　　dp　　　　dq　　　db
　bb　　　　dd　　　　　db　　　pq　　　　　　db

　　　db　　　　　　pq　　　dd　　　pq

　　　　　　pb　　pq　　　dp　　　　　　　　bb

pd　　　　pp　　　qb　　　　　　dq　　　bq

　pb　　　　qb　　　　qd　　　　qp

qq　　　db　　　pq　　bb

Find:　　qq, qp, pp, pd, bd　　　　　　　　　　　**Min.** ___ **Sec.** ___

qq　　　　　　qd　　　　　　pp　　　　db
　　　　　　　　qd
　　　　　　qb　　　　pd　　　　　　　pp
qp　　　　　　　　　qq　　　pq

　　　qq　　　　dd　db　　　　　pp
　　　　　　　　　　　　　　　　　pq

　　　　　　dp　　　　　　　dq　　　　dp

　　pq　　　　　　　　bq
dp　　　bb　　pod　　db
　　pq　　　　　dp　　　　　pd　　　　pp
qb

　　　qq　　　qp　　　　bd　　　　bp
bp　　　pp　　db　　qd　pb

Find:　　bd, bb, dq, dd, pb　　　　　　　　　　　**Min.** ____ **Sec.** ____

Form OM-13
YARDSTICK FIXATIONS

Purpose: Ocular motor, saccadic fixations.

Materials: Wooden yardstick, colored map pins.

Method: Have the child sitting opposite you at a table. Hold the yardstick about 2 feet in front of him as he faces the 18 inch mark. The yardstick will have colored map pins put at various places on it. For example:

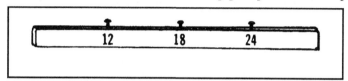

The child will move his eyes quickly from one pin to another in a left to right sequence. Make sure he moves only his eyes. There should not be any head or body movement. Start by having the child do these activities one eye at a time (cover one of his eyes). After he can do each eye individually without any difficulty, have him use both eyes.

Levels 1 to 2:
1. Put the pins at each end and at 12 inches and 24 inches. Have the child move his eyes quickly and accurately from one pin to another in a left to right sequence.
2. Vary the location of the pins. You can use a metronome and every time he hears the beat of the metronome, he moves his eyes.

Levels 3 to 5:
1. Put the pins in various locations on the yardstick. At the beat of the metronome, he is to move his eyes quickly and accurately in a left to right sequence from one pin to another.
2. Vary the position of the yardstick. For example, hold it slightly off center to the right or left, or hold it slightly up or down. He is still to keep his head straight ahead and only move his eyes.

Form OM-14
PENCILS WITH NUMBERS

Purpose: Ocular motor, saccadic fixations.

Materials: Type numbers 1 through 9 on a vertical column on a white piece of paper. Type two columns of the same numbers. Tape these numbers on two pencils. You will also need a metronome for some of these activities.

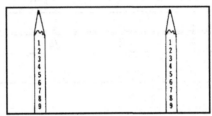

Method: The child is to move his eyes quickly and accurately from one pencil to the other as he holds a pencil in each hand at arm's length. He is to keep his head straight and only move his eyes. Have the child start with one eye at a time (cover the other eye). When you feel each eye is performing at the same level, go to having him do the activities with both eyes. For example:

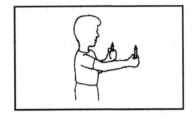

Level 1:
1. At your command, the child is to move his eyes quickly from the top of one pencil to the other.
2. Have him vary the positions of the pencils. For example, one pencil might be 6 inches in front of him and the other at arm's length, or they may be 6 inches apart at arm's length or 3 feet apart at arm's length.

Level 2:
1. At your command, the child is to alternate between the pencils calling out the numbers in sequence from top to bottom. For example, the 1 on the left pencil, then the 1 on the right pencil, 2 on the left pencil, etc.
2. Repeat #1, but vary the positions of the pencils. For example, he can hold the pencils 6 inches apart in front of him or 3 feet apart. He can hold one pencil 1 foot in front of himself and the other at arm's length.
3. Repeat #1 and 2, but have the child call out the numbers to the beat of a metronome.

Level 3: Have the child do Level 2 and then this level.
1. Have the child alternate between pencils by calling out every other number, for example, the 1 on the left pencil, the 2 on the right, the 3 on the left, etc.
2. Repeat #1, but vary the positions of the pencils.
3. Repeat #1 and 2, but use the metronome. Have him call out a number to each beat.

Form OM-14 (continued)
Pencils With Numbers

Levels 4 to 5: Have the child do Levels 2 and 3 and then this level.

1. Have the child alternate between pencils by calling out numbers in sequence starting at the top of one pencil and the bottom of the other. For example, 1 on the left, the 9 on the right, the 2 on the left, the 8 on the right, etc.

2. Repeat #1, but vary the position of the pencils and have him call out the numbers to the beat of a metronome.

Form OM-15
STRING READING

Purpose: To develop proper saccadic fixations going from left to right.

Materials: Typed sheets of paper with letter strings. For example: AA B CC A DD OO P.

Method: The child is to call aloud going from left to right only the single letters. He is not allowed to use his finger to keep his place.

Level 1: Have the strings and letters spaced far apart:
     AA   B   C   DD   O

Level 2: Same as Level 1 but make the spaces slightly closer:
     AA   B   C   DD   O

Levels 3 to 5: Same as Level 2 but vary the lengths of the spaces between the letters:
     AA   O   DD C OO   AA

Space the letters and rows of letters at the same distance as normal reading material.

Form OM-16
NEAR-FAR LETTER NAMING

Purpose: Ocular motor.

Materials: Index cards, marker board.

Method: Type or print letters or numbers on an index card in several rows. Also print some letters or numbers on several rows on the marker board. Have the child do this exercise one eye at a time (cover one of his eyes). When he can do this exercise without difficulty with one eye at a time, have him do it with both eyes at the same time. Have him seated or standing about 15 feet from the board. For Levels 1 and 2, use numbers and spaced far apart. For Levels 3 to 5, use letters and have them spaced closer together.

Levels 1 to 5:
1. Hold the index card about 36 inches in front of his eye. As you slowly move the card toward his eye, he is to call out the letters in a left to right sequence. Stop the card about 6 inches from his eye, quickly remove the card, and have him call out the letters on the board in a left to right sequence. Vary the rows of letters.
2. Vary #1 by having him call out every other letter or every third letter.

Form OM-17

Baseball Fixations

Purpose: Saccadic fixations.

Materials: Marker board.

Method: Have the child stand about 5 feet in front of the board. Draw an X at his eye level. Draw four numbers randomly around the board. For example:

2

3

X

4

1

Levels 2 to 4:

1. Sit facing the child so you can watch his eyes but not block his view of the numbers on the board.
2. The child starts by looking at an X directly in front of him drawn on the board. He is to look at the X, but be aware of the other numbers drawn around it. He is not to move his head or take his eyes off the X.
3. Call out one of the numbers. The child is to move his eyes to that number quickly and accurately. If he does this without looking at any of the other numbers, you give him credit for a hit and he gets to first base.
4. Watch his eyes. If he takes his eyes off the number or looks at you, you call him out.
5. Call out another number. The child now moves his eyes quickly and accurately to that number. If he does it without looking at another number you give him credit and he gets to second base.
6. You continue to watch his eyes. If he takes his eyes off of the number he is supposed to be looking at, call him out.
7. He is to try and get all the way home (this would be four numbers) without getting three outs. You can call the numbers in any random order. You can also use letters instead of numbers.
8. Remember an "out" occurs if he does not look directly at the number you call or if he takes his eyes off of that number before you call the next one.

Form OM-18
SPATIAL ATTENTION

Purpose: To train the transient system and accurate saccadic fixations.

Materials: Marker board.

Method: Have the child do the following activities.

Levels 2 to 5: Have the child stand about 6 feet from the board. Have him look at the X and be aware of the letters surrounding the X. He is not to take his eyes off the X until you call out a letter. He is then to quickly move his eyes to that letter. He should make accurate saccadic fixations and not under- or overshoot the letters. When he has completed his saccadic fixation, have him return his gaze to the X. You can vary the activity by having him keep his eyes on the letter and not go back to the X. Have him start from this letter and you call out the new letter. The following is an example of the board:

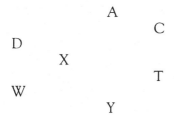

Have the letters spaced so that they present a challenge. Don't put them too close together. You can also vary the number of letters. For Levels 2 and 3, only have a few letters.

Form OM-19
PERIPHERAL TRAINING

Purpose: Train the transient system.

Materials: Span of recognition worksheets, clear plastic sheet with letters.

Method: These activities train peripheral awareness. Peripheral awareness should be stressed with every activity that you do. Always make the child aware of his peripheral vision. In all of these activities, the child should keep his head and eyes straight ahead.

Levels 1 to 2: Stand next to the child and have him stare straight ahead. Hold a familiar object in your hand, e. g., a pencil, set of keys, etc. Slowly move it into his field of vision until he can recognize it.

Level 3:
1. Open a book and have him put his finger on the middle of the page. As he looks at his finger, ask him to see how far to the left and right he can recognize words or letters. The average person should be able to identify at least two letters to the left of the fixation point and four or five on the right.
2. Get a transparency about the size of a sheet of notebook paper. Put a dot in the center and cut out letters of various sizes to paste in various locations around the center dot. Hold the plastic in front of him so that you are looking directly through it at his eyes. Tell him to find and point to certain letters without moving his eyes off of the center dot. Once he can do the entire alphabet, then have him find letter combinations that spell out words. Hold the plastic about 16 inches in front of the child.

Levels 4 to 5:
Use the span of recognition sheets. Start with sheet number one. Have the child stare at the X and tell how many numbers he can see on the left and right of the X. Do sheets two and three next. Make sure he does not move his eyes off of the X. He is only to use his peripheral vision to see the numbers on the side of the X.

Form OM-19 (continued)
PERIPHERAL TRAINING

Span of Recognition 1

7320 X 2549	4832 X 8754
9508 X 3026	7203 X 8402
8674 X 0463	065 X 7013
3658 X 2093	1057 X 2015
9579 X 4802	1098 X 4597
3645 X 8012	3048 X 9734
4026 X 3489	5830 X 8754
7468 X 1804	1574 X 0196
2435 X 9087	8543 X 8590
7539 X 1912	2904 X 1568
1048 X 6371	4872 X 9156
4845 X 9501	380 X 5739
6842 X 5608	1498 X 6903
2465 X 1065	9375 X 0289
3208 X 4960	3412 X 5321
2032 X 8756	087 X 1870
1085 X 7601	4182 X 2308
1208 X 6730	6907 X 4638
9804 X 1645	4902 X 1497

Form OM-19 (continued)
PERIPHERAL TRAINING

Span of Recognition 2

8032 X 6408	8046 X 2308
8146 X 7145	1024 X 4512
1921 X 7539	2084 X 3902
7849 X 5402	6804 X 4068
3860 X 2076	1024 X 8901
4976 X 9794	5648 X 2012
3783 X 9701	7019 X 3852
7102 X 4856	8046 X 0342
1574 X 5982	9013 X 2304
6790 X 1426	3468 X 8421
1036 X 9753	8651 X 3012
9702 X 7407	7654 X 3718
3862 X 7390	7031 X 2987
9074 X 4574	3857 X 9482
3802 X 5015	8352 X 2476
8765 X 6842	2450 X 8632
8042 X 2671	4321 X 8704
3571 X 0932	6453 X 2467
0421 X 7654	9061 X 7430

Form OM-19 (continued)
PERIPHERAL TRAINING

Span of Recognition 3

8759 X 4302	2103 X 6517
2867 X 3402	4902 X 1415
3210 X 3890	1617 X 8010
4902 X 8634	5021 X 0932
0214 X 3905	8472 X 9012
9135 X 2356	0648 X 1045
1047 X 2487	1243 X 2482
1032 X 2913	2163 X 4010
2450 X 1456	6830 X 1912
1041 X 1312	0249 X 6502
4078 X 5890	5863 X 2059
3158 X 6820	1375 X 0492
4921 X 0132	9068 X 3187
6132 X 9856	8146 X 4902
1065 X 2486	1516 X 9101
1097 X 1505	4182 X 4081
3922 X 4721	5976 X 3521
0156 X 3803	0428 X 7632
9568 X 1715	2860 X 5073

Form OM-19 (continued)
PERIPHERAL TRAINING

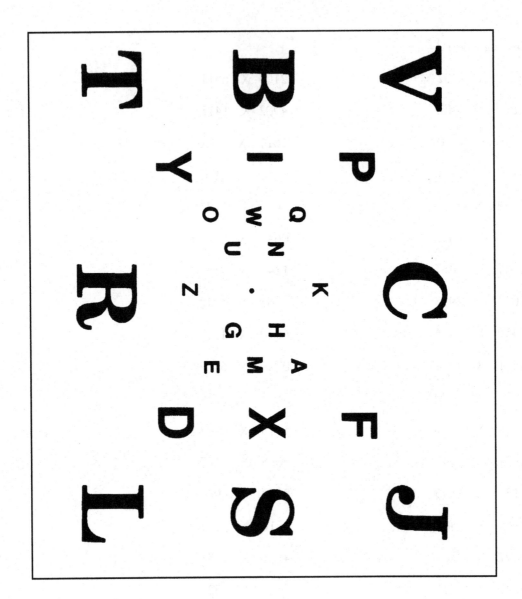

Form OM-20
MARSDEN BALL

Purpose: Ocular motor, smooth pursuit training.

Materials: Marsden ball, letter chart, eye patch. A Marsden ball is a ball hanging on a string.

Method: Have the child keep his eye on the ball at all times. Only in the "Dodge Ball" procedure does he not keep his eyes on the ball. In Levels 1 and 2, he is not to move his head, only his eyes. In all procedures except Levels 1 and 2, hang the ball from the ceiling so that it is at shoulder height and he is standing about 2 feet from it. All children should start with Levels 1 to 2, even older children.

Levels 1 to 2:
1. The child is to lay down on his back with the ball about 2 feet directly over his face. Swing the ball in a left to right direction. The child is to keep his eyes on the ball and not move his head or body. Do not swing the ball too fast or too far out. Do this exercise at first with one of the child's eyes covered with an eye patch. Once he can do each eye individually, have him use both eyes at the same time.
2. Swing the ball left to right, in a circle, diagonally, and head to toe.

Level 3: The child is to hit the ball with his hand while he is standing up. Alternate hands, and have him call out with which hand he is hitting the ball.

Level 4:
1. Dodge Ball: The ball is suspended on a string so the height is just enough to clear the shoulder. The child stands directly under the hook in the ceiling and faces a letter chart. Swing the ball from his front to back on his midline. He must shift his head when the ball swings in front of him to behind him, and when it goes from behind him to his front. For example:

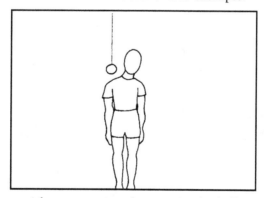

He says a letter on the chart each time it passes his ear. As the ball keeps swinging, it gradually changes its direction and begins to swing from side to side. Do not stop the ball and redirect it. The child continues to read the letters for as long as he can without being hit by the ball.
2. This procedure is "sequencing the Marsden ball". The ball is suspended at a height so that the shoulder can hit it. The two shoulders, elbows, and hands are used to hit the ball. A sequence is given and the child is to say it out loud and then hit the ball with the parts of the body in the proper sequence. For example, "right shoulder", "right hand". Increase the instructions up to six if he can do it.

Level 5: Have the child hit the ball with his hand and stomp the foot on the same side as he hits the ball. Have him call out "right" or "left", depending on which side he is using. When he can do this, have him hit the ball with one hand and stomp the foot on the opposite side. He then calls out the side of the hand and the foot. For example, "right hand, left foot".

Form OM-20 (continued)
MARSDEN BALL

Letter Chart

F	O	D	C	T	P	V	N
B	Y	E	L	Z	K	O	A
T	E	M	K	B	W	F	H
X	B	O	M	S	R	T	F
A	R	X	E	P	V	S	D
P	M	N	B	C	E	A	O
R	C	K	P	E	D	B	G
X	F	A	D	R	S	M	P
M	T	S	G	O	A	X	U
O	H	T	U	K	N	C	S

Form OM-21
VMC Bat

Purpose: Ocular motor.

Materials: VMC (visual motor control) bat, Marsden ball. The VMC bat is a dowel rod about 3 feet long and 1 inch in diameter. It is divided into various colored sections, for example:

r	b	g	g	b	r

Method: Have the Marsden ball hanging in front of the child, chest high. He is to hold the bat horizontally in front of himself with the top of his hands on top of the bat. For example:

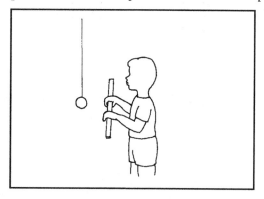

Levels 1 to 2:
1. Have the child hit the ball by pushing the bat at it. See how long he can do it. See how long he can do it without missing the ball.
2. Call out various colors on the bat and have him hit the ball with that color.

Levels 3 to 5:
1. Do Levels 1 to 2.
2. Call out a side and color and have the child hit the ball with that color, e. g., "right red" or "left blue".
3. Have him hit various colors in sequence, e. g., "right red", "left blue", and "right green".
4. Have him hit a number of times with one color and another number of times with another color. For example, ten times with the "right red" and three times with the "left blue". He is not to hit the ball like he would a baseball. Make sure he holds the VMC bat as shown in the method illustration.

Form OM-22
BROCK STRING

Purpose: Saccadic fixations.

Materials: Brock string, metronome.

Method: Levels 1 to 2 are done with a 3 foot length of rough textured string with three large sized colored beads. Levels 3 to 5 are done with an 18 inch length of string between two tongue depressors. Drill a hole near the top of the tongue depressors and put three small colored beads on the string. Tie a knot on the outside of the tongue depressors. For example:

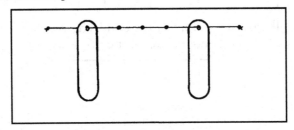

Levels 1 to 2: Tie one end of the string to the top of a chair. The child holds the other end taut against his nose. At your command or at the beat of a metronome, he looks from one bead to the other quickly and accurately. Vary the locations of the beads on the string. Don't put the first bead closer than 5 inches from the child's nose. Have him call the color of the beads as he moves his eyes from one bead to the other. For example:

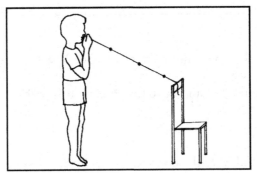

Levels 3 to 5:
1. Do Levels 1 to 2.
2. The child holds one tongue depressor at his nose and the other is held away from his face so that the string is taut. At your command, the child moves his eyes quickly and accurately from one bead to another. You may vary the distance and locations of the beads on the string. Don't have the first bead closer than 5 inches from his nose, for example:

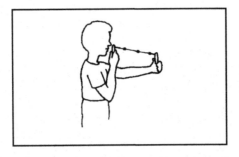

Form OM-22 (continued)
BROCK STRING

3. Have the child do the same as #1, but have him hold the end that is away from his nose in different positions. For example, down and to the right or up and to the left. As you use the metronome, have him move his eyes quickly from bead to bead each time the metronome beats.

Form OM-23
PURSUIT READING

Purpose: Saccadic fixations.

Materials: Reading material to be read for comprehension, walking rail, balance board.

Method: Have the child read the material out loud. If he does not know how to read, have him spell the words. Always have him spell the words in a left to right sequence.

Level 2: Have the child stand and hold the reading material in both hands. Have him move the reading material in circles of varying sizes and in other movement patterns, such as "in and out", "right to left", "up and down", and "diagonally".

Levels 3 to 5: Have the child stand and hold the reading material in both hands. Have him move the reading material in circles and other movement patterns, such as up and down or left and right as he balances on the balance board or walking rail.

Form OM-24
DICTIONARY TRAINING

Purpose: Saccadic fixations.

Materials: Dictionary.

Method: Explain to the child how words are located in a dictionary. Once you feel he has an understanding of this, proceed with the activities.

Level 3: Give the child five words to look up every day. Time him and record his speed of looking up the words.

Levels 4 to 5: Show the child a word with some of its letters left out. He is to use the dictionary to fill in the spaces. For example, w_r_. This could be warm, word, etc. Have him find as many words as he can from the dictionary to fill in these spaces.

Form OM-25
BOARD – BOOK READING

Purpose: To train saccadic fixations.

Materials: Marker board, book.

Method: Copy a paragraph from the child's reading assignment on the board. For Levels 1 and 2, just print letters on the board and on a piece of paper that the child holds.

Levels 1 to 2: The child is to call out the letters on the board and his paper in proper sequence. Both sequences should be same. He does this by alternating between the board and his paper. He will call the first letter from the board, the second from the paper, the third from the board, etc.

Levels 3 to 5: You will put the same paragraph from his book on the board. He is to alternate between the board and the book while he reads aloud. For example, the first word from the paper, the second word from the board.

Form OM-26
ORTHOGRAPHY ACTIVITIES

Purpose: Ocular motor.

Materials: Dictionary.

Method: In English, certain letters occur more frequently in certain positions in words than other letters. This activity is designed to help your child become familiar and pay attention to letter positions in words. For example, in all English words, the letter "T" occurs in the first position more often than any other letter. The following are several lists of letters and their most common position in words. The child should learn the following lists. They are also used for the activities.

Most Common First Letter

First most common	T
Second most common	A
Third most common	W
Fourth most common	H
Fifth most common	S

Most Common Last Letter

First most common	E
Second most common	D
Third most common	T
Fourth most common	S
Fifth most common	R

Most Common First Two Letters

First most common	TH
Second most common	AN
Third most common	WA
Fourth most common	WI
Fifth most common	HI

Most Common Last Two Letters

First most common	HE
Second most common	ND
Third most common	AT
Fourth most common	AS
Fifth most common	ED

Level 3: Have the child look up 10 words that start with each of the most common first two letters. List them below:

1.	6.
2.	7.
3.	8.
4.	9.
5.	10.

Form OM-26 (continued)
ORTHOGRAPHY ACTIVITIES

Level 4: Have the child look up five words that end with each of the most common last two letters. List them below:

1.
2.
3.
4.
5.

Level 5:

1. From the newspaper, have the child find as many words as he can with the most common *first* two letters. Circle the letters. He does not have to write the words down.
2. From the newspaper, have the child find as many words as he can that end with the most common *last* two letters. Circle the letters. He does not have to write them down.

Chapter Five

GROSS MOTOR

"All cognitive mechanisms are based on motor activity."
(Dequiros, 1979)

"We must perceive in order to move, but we must move in order to perceive."
(Piaget, 1948)

Gross Motor Skills and Reading

One of the most controversial and misunderstood areas in the field of learning disabilities is the role of gross motor skills in helping dyslexic children. Most people can understand the importance of studying the role of phonics in reading; however, understanding why a child needs to go through a series of balance activities is much harder to understand. Anyone who has worked with dyslexic children will tell you that a large majority of these children have poor gross motor skills. In fact, one study showed that 95% of dyslexic children had motor instability (Moretti, 2002). The question is why are their gross motor skills usually worse than other children?

Children develop in a normal developmental sequence. Even before birth, the child is developing skills. As early as the fifth gestational month, eye movements are produced by vestibular influences. The child's ability to look at an object, focus, and align his eyes together develops at the end of the second and third postnatal month (Dequiros, 1979). By 5 months, a child's eyes will follow a slowly moving object. When a baby of 6 months hears a noise, he is capable of directing his eyes and head in order to see the object. When he sees it, he tries to grasp it in order to take it to his mouth. By 8 months, he sits independently and creeps on hands and knees and by 12 months, he stands up (Dover, 1979). The first year of crawling, standing up, and walking initiates the development of a new interaction of perceptual modalities that permit him to discover his surrounding environment. During the second year, the influence of gravitational forces produces reinforcement and development of body schemes through experimental walking, falling, and brushing objects. At this stage, a child also develops body awareness and knowledge of his body parts. During the third and fourth years of development, the child has the ability to do a skilled movement with one side of the body while the other side is doing another movement. By the fifth and sixth year, the child has established a preference in using one side of the body over the other (Dequiros, 1979). This is why it is extremely important that a child who has immature motor skills be identified and provided early intervention.

In order to understand how motor activity and development are essential for learning, you need to have some understanding of brain development.

Since creation, the phyletic trend has been toward corticalization of function, i. e., to transfer control of activity from subcortical up to cortical level (Ayres, 1972). As the nervous system developed to meet the expanding needs of existence, the newer structures tended to duplicate older structures and functions and improve upon them rather than devise different functions. Thus the same kinds of function are repeated at several levels of the brain. As they developed, the higher levels remained dependent on the lower structures. The cerebral hemispheres, when they were added, did not provide function that substituted that of the lower brain areas but added abilities that enabled it to deal with the world at a more complex level. The cerebral cortex, which is where our higher cognitive functions such as reading occur, would not be able to interpret sensations that carry information from the environment if it were not for the transmission and processing of the lower brain areas, such as the vestibular system, brainstem, and cerebellum. A child thinks with his whole brain. The educators' error has been in the thinking that all cognitive skills are only cortical, and thus overlooking the probability that some lower brain functions are also critical for these skills (Ayres, 1972). It is the organizing of adaptive responses to environmental demands that has pushed the process of brain development to the point where it is now. The child whose motor skills have not adequately developed is the child who has a higher risk for school failure. If you understand that each developmental step is dependent upon a certain degree of maturation of the previous steps, you will see that reading and language are dependent upon the development of the lower brain areas. As I stated before, the child reads with his whole brain.

Just as the whole brain is concerned with higher brain functions, it is also concerned with more basic functions such as posture and equilibrium; however, in order for the higher brain areas to work efficiently, the lower brain functions must become automatic. If they are not automatic, the higher areas have to assist. This makes the higher functions, such as reading, less efficient. In effect, the higher brain areas become overbooked with body information while trying to correct lower area inadequacies (Dequiros, 1976). The process of being able to exclude body information in order to obtain learning is called *corporal potentiality*. As stated previously, the child develops body awareness during the second year of postnatal life. The next step in normal development is the integration of the postural system, followed by corporal potentiality. Between the age of four and six years, symbolic thought begins to dominate the left cerebral hemisphere. If posture and motor activities are not automatic at this time and the cerebral cortex is forced to be used in these activities, mental actions decrease (Dequiros, 1976). Jackson's law states that "in the case of damage to the central nervous system, functions which appear latest in evolution are lost first" (Dequiros, 1976). For example, in the case of a head injury, the brain will protect its more primitive functions first, such as posture or balance, at the expense of its new functions, such as reading and language. These new functions are not considered as important to the brain as its more primitive and basic functions.

The famous psychologist, Piaget, believed that motor experiences are the foundation of mental development and that all cognitive mechanisms are based on motor activity (Ginsburg, 1969). At the beginning of life, motor activity develops before mental actions, then both work together and coexist, and finally, mental action subordinates motor activity. The premise here is that proper development of motor skills is critical for learning. For a child to have the eye movement skills necessary to keep his eyes on the proper letters in a word when he reads and to be able to have the eye-hand coordination skills necessary to write, his motor skills must be developed to the point of being automatic. This usually comes with normal development. The child, as he matures, develops proper balance and gross motor skills. By gross motor, I mean large muscles such as those used for walking and standing. Development then proceeds from gross to fine motor. Fine motor includes the small muscles like those used for writing. The large muscle groups lying toward the center of the body precede development of the small muscle groups lying at the extremity. Thus total arm precedes elbow, which precedes the wrist, which precedes the fingers, and so forth (Kephart, 1960). This is why we see so many children with learning disabilities who have deficits in coordination, balance, and/or motor skills. This is exhibited not only in gross motor abilities, but also in fine motor, such as visual motor (eye-hand coordination) and ocular motor (eye movement). By having the child use his whole body and move through space, we are training the whole brain. If we just let him sit in front of a computer or try and teach his left and right by clues on his shoes or on his wrists, we are using mainly the higher brain areas. However, if we let the child experience full body movement and both sides of his body through balance and motor activities, then we are training the whole brain, including the lower levels.

In order to explain two important systems for learning, I will start with the vestibular system. The inner ear has auditory and nonauditory organs. The cochlea is the auditory organ dedicated to hearing, while the vestibular apparatus (also called the labyrinth) is the nonauditory organ dedicated to posture, equilibrium, muscular tones, and spatial orientation. The vestibular apparatus also controls the movements of the eyes (through the vestibular-oculomotor pathways) and many other functions connected with intentional and coordinated movements (Dequiros, 1979). To emphasize the importance of this system, the vestibular nerve is the first among all sensory nerves to be myelinated. Within each vestibular apparatus are three semicircular canals that are endolymph-filled ducts oriented at right angles to each other so that they represent all three planes in space. The most efficient stimuli to the semicircular canals are angular transient

(short-term) and fast (high frequency) head movements of at least 2 degrees per second. When the head moves at slower speeds, the endolymph, cupula, and hair cells all move at the same speed as the head (Fisher, 1991). The functional implication for treatment is that any head position or head movement will result in stimulation of some combination of vestibular receptor cells. Planning, therefore, should give consideration to activities that provide stimuli: 1) in all body (head) positions and in all planes of three dimensional space, 2) that vary in speed from static (not moving) to fast, 3) that are linear and angular, and 4) that are transient and sustained (Fisher, 1991).

Balance and spatial orientation are maintained by streams of afferent impulses that are generated by the ocular system, the vestibular system, and the proprioceptors (muscles, joints, viscera, and skin). The proprioceptive impulses of the muscles and tendons, and especially of the joints of the neck, are extremely important. Regulatory systems in the brain and spinal nervous structures act like computers, taking the constant stream of impulses from the eyes, ears, and proprioceptive senses, regulating them to constantly alert the body to maintain balance in its normal position. Thus, these sense organs provide a running commentary on both the external and internal environment of the individual, from which the central nervous system collects an integrated pattern that maintains both equilibrium and spatial orientation (Levinson, 1980). A dysfunction of the vestibular system alone, or in combination with its integrating and regulating computer, the cerebellum, may well account not only for the motor imbalance and spatial incoordination noted in dyslexia, but also for the visual, auditory, proprioceptive, and directional dyscoordination as well (Levinson, 1980).

One procedure that you can use on a child to test for these dysfunctions is the Rhomberg Test. This test is used to see if a child with his eyes closed, and only using vestibular and proprioceptive inputs, can maintain his balance. Have the child stand with his feet together, his arms hanging at his side and both eyes closed. If he moves his feet apart this may indicate a cerebellar disturbance or immaturity. If he sways back and forth, this may indicate a difficulty with proprioceptive information (Dequiros, 1976).

When we look at something, the light enters our eyes through the pupil and focuses on the back part of the eye (retina). In order to see clearly, the light must focus on a small pitted area called the fovea. This is only 1.5 mm in diameter and has cones in the center to yield high visual acuity. If the light does not focus on this area, your vision is blurred. There are six extraocular muscles that move each eye—four rectus and two oblique. When you move your eyes, they move at a very high rate of speed. What makes this very complicated is that both of your eyes must focus on the same thing at the exact same time. If one eye

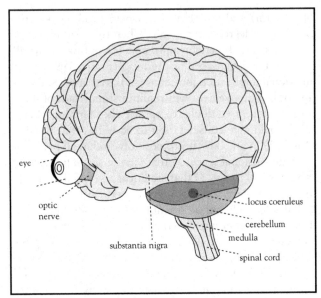

Figure 5-1. Side view of the human brain showing the location of the cerebellum.

is off just a fraction of a second, your vision is blurred or you see double. Therefore, if you have your head turned sideways, one eye will have to travel further than the other eye. This requires incredible precision. To give you an idea how precise the coordination of the extraocular muscles must be, let me give you an example of the coordination of other muscles. Several years ago, researchers determined what it takes for 10 healthy male softball players to hit a target 3 meters away by throwing tennis balls at it. Coils taped to the men's fingers, hands, and arms relayed joint positions to a computer when a microswitch on their middle finger was triggered as soon as they released the ball. To hit the target, the researchers found, a thrower had to open his fingers to release the ball within a particular 2 msec timeframe in the course of his throwing movement. The subjects often missed because their release times varied by as little as 10 msec (Wickelgren, 1998).

It is obvious that something has to act as a computer and coordinate the timing of these complicated movements. Something has to accurately move your eyes when you read, determine how much pressure to put on your pencil when you write, and where to aim your toothbrush so that it goes into your mouth and not your eye. The area of the brain that is responsible for this is the cerebellum (Figure 5-1).

One of the early advocates of the idea that the function of the cerebellum might be related to dyslexia was Harold Levinson, MD. He published his book, *A Solution to the Riddle Dyslexia*, in 1980. He discovered that 75% of the dyslexic cases he analyzed contained past or present developmental evidence of balance, coordination, and rhythmic motor disturbances. The symptoms of dyslexics

he studied included:

1. Instability of letters and words.
2. Words, syllables, and letters were often inappropriately inserted during reading.
3. Words, syllables, letters and parts of letters were frequently skipped over and omitted.
4. Letters and syllables of successive words were periodically fused or condensed and read as new words: "the cat", for example, might be read as "that".
5. Omitted letters, syllables and words were often displaced to more distant parts of the same sentence or paragraph.
6. Reading errors characterized by omission, insertion, displacement, condensation, rotation, reversals, substitution, and guessing tendencies.
7. Active and conscious letter, word, and sentence movement.
8. Sloppy and disorganized writing. Dyslexic children often reposition their heads, bodies and arms while angling the paper as if they are searching for a comfortable position.
9. Sequential and single types of memory disturbances for sensory, motor, temporal, and directional events.
10. Ocular motor tracking difficulties.

Levinson assumes that there exists a cerebellum-vestibular determined ocular motor dysmetria or nystagmus (a rapid involuntary movement of the eye, usually in the horizontal direction) in dyslexia, and this nystagmus secondarily scrambles the visual input. It scrambles the temporal-spatial sequence of the visual input at the retinal site. According to his reading hypotheses, dyslexics have a subclinical nystagmus with a related ocular fixation and sequential tracking dysfunction caused by a cerebellum – vestibular dysfunction. This makes it very difficult for dyslexics to accurately track their eyes as they read. A good analogy for this is the firing system on a moving ship. It has to have a stable platform in order to accurately fire and hit a target (Levinson, 1980).

The cerebellum is the size of a baseball and is bean shaped. It is in the back of our skull, perched upon the brainstem, and has more than 100 billion neurons (Wickelgren, 1998). This is more neurons than the remainder of the brain combined (Allen, 1997). It is physiologically connected with all major subdivisions of the central nervous system, including the cerebrum, basal ganglia, diencephalon, limbic system, brainstem, and spinal cord by monosynaptic or multisynaptic pathways. It is, therefore, one of the busiest intersections in the human brain. Nonetheless, for more than a century, neurologists and neuroscientists alike have held the view that the singular function of the human cerebellum is to help coordinate movement (Allen, 1997).

For over a century, the cerebellum has been regarded by the scientific community as a motor organ. Recent studies now show that the cerebellum is instrumental in nonmotor activities such as: 1) judging the timing of events, and 2) solving perceptual and spatial reasoning problems (Gao, 1996). Evidence suggests the involvement of the cerebellum in cognitive functions such as language, spatial and temporal elaboration, learning, and planning (Silveri, 1994). The role of the cerebellum in timed sequential cognitive processing may be analogous to its role in motor processing and suggests a mechanism by which cognitive events become sequentially and temporally labeled (Schmahmann, 1997). This view is best supported by positron emission tomography (PET). This procedure showed activation in the inferior and lateral part of the cerebellum during a rule-based, word generated task (Kim, 1994). The lateral most portion of the cerebellum is also involved in voluntary motor control (Ito, 1990).

The importance of the cerebellum to human growth is proven by the fact that it has enlarged between threefold and fourfold in only the past million years (Levinson, 1980). The increase in size of the dentate nucleus of the cerebellum is paralleled by an increase in size of the cortical area influenced by cerebellar output. This area at the same time showed an expansion of cerebellar function to include involvement in some language and cognitive skills. The dentate nucleus exerts its influence by projecting via the thalamus to the cerebral cortex. The regions of the cerebellum concerned with the generation of eye movements are connected with primary motor and premotor areas of the cerebral cortex (Kim, 1994). Cerebellar activation has also been reported to be highest in the early stages of learning novel information or when nonmotor and motor sequences of information must be processed (Allen, 1997).

The two major anatomical compartments of the cerebellum are the cortex and deep nuclei. Purkinje cells, the only outputs from the cerebellum project through inhibitory connections to the deep cerebellar nuclei which provides the output to other brain regions. Inputs are transmitted to the cerebellum over climbing fibers and mossy fibers. The climbing fibers arise from the olivary nuclei and the mossy fibers from the brainstem (Raymond, 1996).

All of the knowledge of the cerebellum that has been acquired has shown that we now know the cerebellum is not just involved in motor skills. Cerebellum functions include:

1. The regulation of the rate, force, rhythm, and accuracy of movements (Schmahmann, 1991).
2. The memory storage for motor learning (Shadmehr, 1997).
3. Regulating the timing of learned movements (Raymond, 1996).
4. Linkage with Broca's language area allows it to be involved in the acquisition of language.
5. Involvement in the acquisition of phonological skills (Fisher, 1991).
6. Involvement in spatial dysgraphia (Moretti, 2002).
7. Timing of various muscle contractions to ensure the speed and accuracy of maneuver (Wickelgren, 1998).
8. Controlling precise temporal interplay between different sets of muscles (Silveri, 1994).
9. Involvement in spatial learning.
10. The execution of visual tracking.
11. Parts of the cerebellum are activated by the generation of verbs to go with nouns (but not nouns to go with verbs).
12. Coordination between eye position and hand/arm movement.
13. Visual motor coordination.
14. Helping with attention.
15. Mental imagery.
16. Influence in working memory.
17. Influence in linguistic processing.
18. Influence in emotional states.
19. Involved in the timing that is involved in perception.
20. Attention shifting (Schmahmann, 1997).

Symptoms of children with a cerebellar – vestibular dysfunction include:

1. Ocular fixation difficulty.
2. Visual-motor difficulty.
3. Difficulty catching, throwing, and kicking.
4. Visual-spatial or perceptual difficulty.
5. Awkward holding of pencil.
6. Clumsy and/or awkward coordination.
7. Difficulty with fine motor coordination.
8. Graphomotor incoordination, i. e., poor letter formation and spacing (Levinson, 1980).

The most common theory in the cause of dyslexia is the *Phonological Deficit Hypothesis*. This states that the neurological abnormalities in the language areas around the Sylvian fissure lead to failure to develop phonological awareness skills at the age of 5, thereby interfering with the learning of phoneme-grapheme and grapheme-phoneme conversions (phonics), which are critical requirements in learning to read. There is evidence that phonological awareness deficits persist through life and that training of at-risk children on phonological awareness leads to acquisition of reading (Fawcett, 2001). No one disputes that phonics is an important piece of the puzzle in dyslexics; however, if it was strictly a phonics problem, why would most dyslexic children also have difficulties in ocular motor, motor skills, balance (Fawcett, 1999), and visual motor (Jones, 1999) areas? Obviously, there is more to dyslexia than just phonics. In one study of dyslexic children, 97% showed evidence of a cerebellar-vestibular dysfunction (Frank, 1973). In another study, 95% showed statistically significant impairment in cerebellar tests with deficits on postural stability and muscle tone (Moretti, 2002). This is why there are now several other theories on dyslexia in addition to the Phonological Deficit Hypothesis. These include the Magnocellar Deficit Hypothesis, the Double Deficit Hypothesis, and the Cerebellar Deficit Hypothesis. The Double Deficit Hypothesis states that dyslexic children have difficulties in the speed of processing almost all stimuli and that dyslexia is characterized by both phonological and naming speed *core* deficits. The Cerebellar Deficit Hypothesis states that children with dyslexia show a range of cerebellar signs. These include articulatory difficulties (and hence, phonological problems), slowed central processing speed, and deficits in motor skills. This theory states that reading is severely impaired because it depends on two aspects of cerebellar function: learning new skills and becoming expert in these skills (Fawcett, 2001).

This section on the cerebellum is not intended to claim that the cerebellum is the cause of dyslexia; however, it should be considered as a possible participant in dyslexia. Therefore, a training program must include activities that activate the cerebellum as well as vestibular function.

Tips for a Successful Gross Motor Therapy Program

In order to have a successful therapy program, you need to provide the child with a flood of sensory motor experiences. This would include gross motor and fine motor movements that stimulate visual, tactile, and kinesthetic awareness. Especially evident from research is the importance of the use of the visual modality, such as activities involving eye-hand and eye-foot correlation activities. Parents need to be aware that gross motor activities should begin before age of 2 with such activities as climbing, walking, running, jumping, and kicking. These activities help stimulate the general wiring patterns of these behaviors. Gross motor activities help provide the brain with its chief energy source—glucose. In essence, these activities increase blood flow, which feeds the brain and may increase normal connections during this critical period (Gabbard, 1993).

The following are important procedures that should be incorporated in a gross motor program:

1. A powerful tool that can be used with a gross motor therapy program and other programs as well is *mental imagery*. Mental imagery is the process of mentally recreating an experience by using images and a variety of senses. It has been shown in many studies that imagery plays a role in motor skills. Imagining one's own body movements lights up many of the same brain areas as actual performance of these movements (Bracke-Tolkmitt, 1989). It has been demonstrated that it takes almost the same time to perform an actual motor task as to mentally simulate the same performance. This suggests that central neuronal mechanisms responsible for performance of a given type of motor activity are also utilized during simulation of the same movements. Mental imagery causes the regional blood flow to increase in the frontal lobes, especially in the premotor cortex and the supplementary motor area (Delety, 1990). It has been found that the use of imagery along with physical practice enhances performance more than the use of physical practice without imagery. Mental imagery has two basic cognitive approaches—internal and external. *Internal imagery* is where the performer visualizes the skill as if he was actually performing it and observing through his own eyes. In contrast, *external imagery* is where the performer visualizes himself as if watching from the outside (as if observing oneself on film). Motor tasks seem to be more receptive to internal imagery. However, it has been suggested that a combination of both internal and external is the most effective way of improving performance (Moretti, 2002). When you use mental imagery with a child (Pie, 1996):

   a) Describe in detail what the child should "see" and "feel" when performing.

   b) It is useful to begin your imagery sessions with some deep breathing or other relaxation.

   c) The sessions should be 3 to 5 minutes.

   d) It should complement rather than replace actual physical practice.

   e) Just as one teaches physical skills in a progressive manner, it is helpful to begin with simple static images. For example, image a soccer ball before attempting to rehearse more complex images like kicking it.

f) Advanced imagery can include having them image changing the color or orientation of an object (E, 2001).

2. Do activities that train cerebellar and vestibular areas:

a.) Balance activities.

b.) Activities that deal in spatial and temporal skills, for example, knot tying or putting beads in the right sequence on a string.

c.) Activities that involve dual tasks, for example, balance and vision. An example would be walking on the walking rail and calling out letters on a chart hanging on the wall.

d.) Activities that require sequencing involving several parts of the body.

e.) Activities that require timing, for example, activities that require a metronome.

f.) Activities that use ocular motor skills.

g.) Activities that require visual-motor coordination.

References

Allen, G. (1997). Attentional activation of the cerebellum independent of motor involvement. *Science, 275*(5308), 1940-1943.

Ayres, J. A. (1972). *Sensory integration and learning disorders.* Los Angeles, CA: Western Psychological Services.

Bracke-Tolkmitt, R. (1989). The cerebellum contributes to mental skills. *Behavioral Neuroscience, 103,* 442-446.

Delety, J. (1990). The cerebellum participates in mental activity: Tomographic measurements of regional cerebral blood flow. *Brain Research, 535,* 313-317.

Dequiros, J. B. (1976). Diagnosis of vestibular disorders in the learning disabled. *Journal of Learning Disabilities, U9,* 50-56.

Dequiros, J. B. (1979). *Neuropsychological fundamentals in learning disabilities* (rev ed.). Novato, CA: Academic Therapy Publications.

Dover, W. (1979). Developmental motor responses by age. *Journal of Optometric Vision Development, 10*(4).

E, S. (2001). Using mental imagery to enhance children's motor performance. *Journal of Physical Education, Recreation and Dance, 72*(2), 19-23.

Fawcett, A. J. (2001). Cerebellar tests differentiate between groups of poor readers with and without iq discrepancy. *Journal of Learning Disabilities, 34,* 119.

Fawcett, A. J. (1999). Performance of dyslexic children on cerebellar and cognitive tests. *Journal of Motor Behavior, 31,* 68-78.

Fisher, A. G. (1991). *Sensory integration theory and practice.* Philadelphia: F. A. Davis Company.

Frank, J. (1973). Dysmetric dyslexia and dyspraxia. *Journal of the American Academy of Child Psychiatry, 4,* 690-701.

Gabbard, C. (1993). Windows of opportunity for early brain and motor development. *Journal of Physical Education, Recreation and Dance, 69*(8), 54-55.

Gao, J. H. (1996). Cerebellum implicated in sensory acquisition and discrimination rather than motor control. *Science, 272*(5261), 545-547.

Ginsburg, O. H. (1969). *Piaget's theory of intellectual development.* New York: Prentice-Hall.

Ito, M. (1990). A new physiological concept on cerebellum. *Revue Neurologique, 146,* 564-569.

Jones, J. (1999). Dyslexia may be associated with cerebellar abnormalities. *British Medical Journal, 318*(7195), 1372.

Kephart, N. L. (1960). *The slow learner in the classroom.* Columbus, OH: Charles E. Merrill Books.

Kim, S. G. (1994). Activation of a cerebellar output nucleus during cognitive processing. *Science, 265*(5174), 949-951.

Lane, K. A. (1988). *Reversal errors, theories and therapy procedures.* Santa Ana, CA: Vision Extension.

Levinson, H. (1980). *A solution to the riddle dyslexia.* New York: Springer-Verlag.

Moretti, R. (2002). Peculiar aspects of reading and writing performances in patients with olivopontocerebellar atrophy. *Perceptual and Motor Skills, 94,* 677-694.

Piaget, J. (1948). *The child's conception of space.* London: Routledge and Kegan Paul, Ltd.

Pie, J. (1996). Imagery orientation and vividness: Their effect on a motor skill performance. *Journal of Sport Behavior, 19*(1), 32-49.

Raymond, J. L. (1996). The cerebellum: A neuronal learning machine. *Science, 272*(5265), 1126-1131.

Shadmehr, R. (1997). Neural correlate of motor memory consolidation. *Science, 277*(5327), 821-825.

Schmahmann, J. D. (1991). An emerging concept: The cerebellar contribution to higher function. *Archives of Neurology, 48,* 1178-1210.

Schmahmann, J. D. (1997). *The cerebellum and cognition.* New York: Academic Press.

Silveri, M. C. (1994). The cerebellum contributes to linguistic production. *Neurology,* 2047-2050.

Wickelgren, I. (1998). The cerebellum: The brain's engine of agility. *Science, 281*(5383), 1588-1590.

Form GM-I
ONE FOOT HOP

Purpose: Gross motor.

Materials: None.

Method: Have the child do the following activities.

Level 1:
1. Have the child hop in place on one leg, hop four steps forward, four steps backward, hop to the left, hop to the right, hop in place and turn around.
2. Repeat with opposite foot.

Level 2:
1. Hop while grasping the ankle with the opposite hand behind the back.
2. Hop while grasping the leg in front of the body with both hands.
3. The child should try to do at least 10 hops across the room on each foot.

Form GM-2
STEPPING STONES

Purpose: Gross motor.

Materials: Different colored tile or carpet cut into 4-inch squares (have 20 squares—10 of one color and 10 of another color), metronome.

Method: The child is to walk on the squares. He is to keep his body straight and have good posture.

Level 1: Put the squares in a straight line. The child is to walk on them and keep his balance.

Level 2:
1. Arrange the squares slightly off center with one color on the right of center and the other on the left of center. For example:

R	B
R	B
R	B

   Have the child walk on the squares and call out the side that is stepping on the square. For example, each time he steps on the blue square, he calls out "right" and each time he steps on the red square, he calls out "left".
2. Put the squares in various patterns that make up letters or numbers. Have the child walk on the patterns and tell you which letter or number it is.

Form GM-3
HEEL AND TOE ROCK

Purpose: Gross motor.

Materials: None.

Method: Have the child do the following activities while he is standing with his feet together and his arms hanging at his side.

Level 1:
1. Rise on his toes for three counts, lower his heels, and lift his toes for three counts.
2. Rock back and forth, holding each balance position for three counts.
3. Have him hold his balance for longer periods of time.
4. Do the same activities but have him do them with his arms folded in front of his chest.

Level 2: Same as Level 1, but the child does the activities with his eyes closed. Only do these activities for three counts.

Form GM-4
Pattern Hopping

Purpose: Gross motor, laterality.

Materials: None.

Method: The child will do the following activities.

Level 1:
1. The child stands in front of you, arms at his side. Have him hop up and down. Make sure both his feet leave and touch the floor at the same time.
2. Have him hop across the room on one foot. Have him do it first with his right foot and then hop back on his left foot.

Level 2:
1. Clap a pattern and have him hop to the pattern. For example, one clap, pause and two quick claps would be one hop, pause and two quick hops. Have him do this first on both feet, then on one foot.
2. Do #1, but have the child facing away from you so he cannot see you clapping.

Level 3: Have the child facing you. Clap a pattern. He is to alternate feet as he hops to the pattern. For example, clap, clap, pause, clap, clap, clap would be right, left, pause, right, left, right.

Level 4: Have the child facing away from you. Clap a pattern. He is to alternate feet and call out which foot he is hopping on as he hops to the pattern. For example, clap, pause, clap, clap, he would hop and call out "right", pause, "left", "right".

Form GM-5
Gross Motor Balance Sequencing

Purpose: Gross motor.

Materials: None.

Method: Have the child do the following activities.

Level 1:
1. Have the child assume a hand and knee position on the floor. Have him raise one hand in the air. The goal is to maintain his balance for a count of ten. Do the same but have him raise the other hand in the air.
2. Repeat #1, but have the child raise a leg instead of a hand.
3. Repeat #1, raising hand and leg on the same side of body.
4. Repeat #1, raising hand and leg on opposite sides of body.

Level 2:
1. Have the child balance on his tiptoes for a count of ten.
2. Have him rise smoothly and evenly from a sitting position on the floor while keeping his arms folded on his chest.
3. Have him maintain his balance while walking forward and backward on his knees.
4. Have him maintain his balance for a count of ten while standing on one foot. (For children 6 and under, maintain balance for a count of five.)

Level 3:
1. Have him maintain his balance while hopping on one foot with his eyes closed. Repeat with other foot.
2. Have him maintain his balance while jumping with both feet with his eyes closed. He is to make 1/4 or 1/2 turns while jumping.
3. Repeat #2, but he is to use only one foot. Repeat with other foot.

Levels 4 to 5:
1. Have the child stand and maintain his balance while moving his arm and leg on the same side of his body. His arm and leg are to be kept straight and pivoted from the shoulder and hip in an arc to the side.
2. Repeat # 1, but have him use his arm and leg on the opposite side of his body.

Form GM-6
FOOT TAPPING

Purpose: To train rhythm, sequential motor skills, laterality.

Materials: Metronome.

Methods: Have the child take his shoes and socks off.

Level 1: Tell the child that each time he hears the metronome, he is to tap his right foot (you point to the foot). Vary the foot and the speed of the metronome.

Level 2: Same as Level 1, but at each beat of the metronome, he switches feet.

Level 3:
1. Work on sequencing. For example, at each beat, do the following sequence: three times with the right foot then three times left foot. Continue switching back and forth.
2. Go up to three instructions. For example, three times with the right foot, two times with the left foot, and three times together.

Level 4: Work up to four instructions. For example, three times with the right foot, two times with the left foot, two times together, and four times with the right foot.

Level 5: Instead of the metronome you will clap. Do up to four instructions, but he is not to tap until he hears you clap.

Form GM-7
BEAN BAG BASKETBALL

Purpose: Gross motor.

Materials: Bean bags, trash can, balance rail.

Method: Put a trash can or bucket at various distances from the child.

Level 1: He is to try and throw the bean bag into the can. Have him use one hand at a time then both hands together. He can throw over- or underhand.

Level 2:
1. Have the child stand on the end of the walking rail in a heel to toe position. Have him keep his balance and throw the bean bags into the can. He can throw either over- or underhand. Have him do it first with his right hand, then his left hand, and finally both hands at the same time. Keep score of how many baskets he makes.
2. Have the child stand about 10 feet in front of the trash can. Have him close his eyes and see if he can throw the bean bag into the can. Keep his score.

Form GM-8
CRAWLING ACTIVITIES

Purpose: Gross motor.

Materials: None.

Method: Do these activities with the child lying on his stomach or on his back. Have him keep his head up and look straight ahead (if he is on his back have him look straight up at the ceiling).

Levels 1 and 2: Have him slide his body along the floor by using only his arms and dragging his legs, or only his shoulders and legs and dragging his arms. For example:

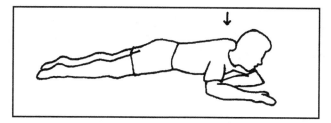

Have him use only his hips and shoulder motion and drag his arms and legs. For example:

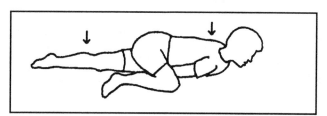

Form GM-9
MARINE CRAWL

Purpose: Gross motor.

Materials: None.

Method: Child is to be on his stomach with his eyes looking at a target across the room. At your command, he is to crawl forward on his stomach toward the target without taking his eyes off of it. He is to crawl in such a way that he is pulling with his arm on one side of the body and pushing with his leg on the other side. The target can be anything—a chair or a toy, etc.

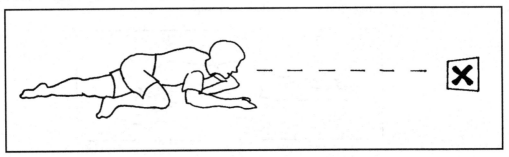

Observations: He is to keep his eyes on the target.

Levels 1 and 2: Have him crawl forward toward the target. Make sure he has good form and is pulling with his arm on one side and pushing with his leg on the other side.

Levels 3 to 5: Same as Level 1, but have him also crawl backwards away from the target. For this, he will have to push with his arm and bring his opposite leg up to his side.

Form GM-10
CREEPING ACTIVITIES

Purpose: Gross motor.

Materials: Metronome.

Method: All these procedures are done on hands and knees. For example:

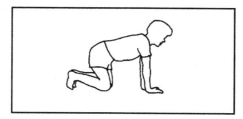

The procedures can be done with either head leading (going forward) or with feet leading (going backward). Each procedure is done in various sequence patterns of hands and knees leaving and touching the ground. Use the following codes for the patterns: LG = leaves ground, TG = touches ground, H = hand, K = knee.

Use the following patterns:
A. Moving the hands and knees on the same side of the body, for example, right hand then right knee.

1st Movement	2nd Movement	3rd Movement	4th Movement
1. HLG	2. KLG	3. HTG	4. KTG

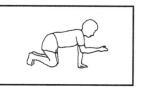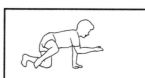

2. KLG	HLG	KTG	HTG
3. H & K	LG	H & K	TG

B. Moving the hands and knees on the opposite sides of the body, for example, left knee then right hand.

1. HLG	KLG	HTG	KTG
2. KLG	HLG	KTG	HTG
3. H & K	LG	H & K	TG

Level 1: At a slow pace, have the child practice the pattern in sequences of A & B above. Only go forward.

Level 2: At a slow pace, have the child practice the pattern sequences A & B above, going forward and backward.

Level 3: Using a metronome, have the child do the pattern sequences A & B above, going forward and backward to the beat of the metronome. He makes one move for each beat of the metronome.

Levels 4 to 5: Using a metronome, have the child do the pattern sequence A & B above going forward and backward to the beat of the metronome. He is to call out which hand or knee he is lifting off the floor. For example, "right hand" or "left knee".

Form GM-11
COLORED SQUARES

Purpose: Gross motor, laterality.

Materials: Carpet squares, tile squares or plastic squares, metronome.

Method: Arrange a large pattern of colored squares on the floor. For example:

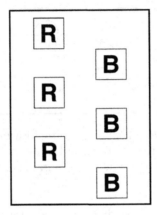

Color code the child's feet, one color for each foot. For example, his right foot is coded red and his left foot blue.

Level 2: Have him walk through the colored squares only on those that match his color coded feet. For example, tell him that his right foot is blue and his left foot is red. Vary the codes for his feet.

Level 3:
1. Have the child hop one foot at a time on the squares that are the same color as the colors coded for his feet. For example, code his left foot blue. He is to hop only on the blue squares with his left foot.
2. Code each foot and have him hop alternating between feet to the correct color.
3. Add a metronome. Each time he hears the metronome beat, he will alternate feet and hop to a different square. Make sure he only hops on the square that is the same color as the color you assigned to his foot.

Levels 4 to 5:
1. Tell the child the sequence you want him to hop. For example, hop three times on the right foot and two on the left. Each time he hears the metronome beat, he will hop to the colored square that is the same color as the color that his foot is coded.
2. Vary the color code for the feet and the sequences. For example:

```
R    G    R    G
R    G    R
G    R    G    R
G    R    G
```

Form GM-12
HEAD TILT

Purpose: Vestibular stimulation.

Materials: None.

Method: The child tilts his head while he keeps his eyes on a target.

Level 1: Have the child look at a target. Have him walk around the room or kneel down without taking his eye off of the target.

Level 2:
1. With the child's eyes closed, have him practice bending his head to the positions you call out. For example, right shoulder, left shoulder, etc. After each instruction, he is to bring his head to the starting position before he does the next instruction.
2. Have him do the same thing with his eyes open.

Level 3: Same as Level 2 but vary the positions of the child. For example, seated, standing, on all fours.

Level 4: Same as Levels 2 and 3, but:
1. The child looks at you and copies the direction you go. When you bend your head to the right shoulder, the child bends his head to his left.
2. You do several positions before he does them. He is to copy them from memory.

Level 5: Same as Level 4 but he bends his head to the same shoulder you do. For example, you bend to your right, he bends to his right shoulder.

Form GM-13
EIGHT SQUARE BOUNCING

Purpose: Develop gross motor skills.

Materials: Colored squares.

Yellow	Red	Green
Black	Space	White
Purple	Blue	Orange

The child stands on the "space" square and has a ball that he can bounce. Have him face the red square.

Level 1: Starting at the red square, bounce the ball five times in each square moving right and going in a clockwise direction. The child can use both of his hands. Practice to complete this in a continuous manner without stopping (if possible). Then, do the same going left.

Level 2: Same as Level 1, but the child only uses one hand.

Level 3: Same as Levels 1 and 2, but the child uses his nondominant hand.

Levels 4 and 5:
1. Same as Levels 2 and 3, but alternate right and left hands.
2. Vary how many times you want the child to bounce the ball.
3. Call out which square and hand you want him to use. For example, bounce four times on the red square with your left hand, then three times on the orange square with your right hand.

Form GM-14
LETTER TRACKING AND BOUNCING A BALL

Purpose: Gross motor, laterality.

Materials: Letter chart, playground ball.

Method: Have the child slowly walk towards a letter chart hung at his eye level on the wall about 15 feet from him.

Level 1: As he walks toward the chart, he calls out a letter with each step he takes. Have him call out the letters in a left to right sequence. If he doesn't know his letters yet, he takes a step each time you call out and point to a letter.

Level 2:
1. As he walks toward the chart, have him call out the leg he is stepping out on before he calls out the letter. For example, "right leg" then the letter.
2. Have the child bounce a ball as he takes a step and calls out a letter. Have him call out the letters in a left to right sequence. Start by having him just use his right hand and then his left. Have him bounce the ball once for each letter.
3. Alternate between the right and left hands and have him call out which hand he is bouncing the ball with before he calls out the letter.

Levels 3 and 4: Have the child bounce a ball as he takes a step and calls out a letter. Have him call out the letters in a left to right sequence. Vary the number of times he bounces the ball with each hand before he calls out the hand and the letter. For example, one bounce with the right hand as he steps out with his right leg. He then calls out "right" and names the letter. Next have him bounce the ball two times with his left hand as he steps out with his left leg. He then calls out "left" and names a letter. He continues with this sequence until you tell him to stop.

Letter Chart

F O D C T P V N

B Y E L Z K O A

T E M K B W F H

X B O M S R T F

A R X E P V S D

P M N B C E A O

R C K P E D B G

X F A D R S M P

M T S G O A X U

O H T U K N C S

Form GM-15
ACTIVITIES FOR BALL BOUNCING

Purpose: Gross motor, laterality.

Materials: Playground ball (ball about 4 to 5 inches in diameter that has a good bounce), colored tape, metronome.

Method: Have the child do the following activities.

Level 1: Have the child use one or both hands, whatever is comfortable. Put the child in a sitting position. Have him bounce the ball between his legs. Begin with small, gentle bounces and increase vigor.

Level 2: Alternating hands while standing still:
1. Begin with ball in right hand. Bounce it close to the feet and in front. As the ball rebounds, force it down again with left hand. Bounce the ball, alternating hands as long as possible.
2. Begin different rhythmic patterns of ball bouncing. For example, start with ball in left hand. As it rebounds from the floor, use this pattern: 2R, 1 Both, 2L, 1 Both, 2R. Some other patterns could be: 2 Both, 1L, 3R, 3L, or 1R, 2 Both, 2L, 1R, 2 Both.
3. Complete #1 and 2 while walking.
4. Use different degrees of force while standing still or moving.
5. Create different walking patterns.

Level 3: Have the child alternate hands as he does these activities:
1. Make three 48-inch circles from colored tape on the floor. For example, red, green, and blue. The child must bounce the ball within the restricted circle. Each circle is coded. For example, blue indicates bouncing with both hands, red indicates right hand, and green indicates left hand. The child moves from each circle, changing activity according to the code.
2. Make three 30-inch squares from colored tape on the floor. For example, white, black, and yellow. The child must bounce the ball within the square according to each color's particular code. White indicates an alternating hand bounce: R, L, R, L. Black indicates the pattern: 1 both hands, 2L, 2R, 1 both hands. Yellow indicates the pattern: 1L, 2R, 1 both hands.
3. On the floor are 30-inch x 15-inch rectangles that are divided in half to make two 15-inch squares. Child stands in one 15-inch square and bounces the ball within the limits of the other 15-inch square. Use various patterns starting with simple to complex. For example:
    a. As many as possible with both hands
    b. As many as possible with left hand
    c. As many as possible with right hand
    d. Alternating L, R, L, R, L
    e. Both hands, 2L, 2R, 1L, 2 both.

Levels 4 and 5:
1. Same as Level 3, but a metronome is added. Set the pattern to a constant rhythm by use of a metronome. Child bounces the ball each time the metronome beats.
2. Create a course with different squares, circles, lines. Include places where child doesn't bounce the ball, but hops. For example, in all triangle shapes he holds the ball and hops on one foot; in square shapes, he holds the ball and hops on both feet.

Form GM-16
BEANBAG ACTIVITIES

Purpose: Gross motor.

Materials: Beanbags.

Method: Tell the child to do the following activities.

Level 1:
1. Throw the beanbag up in the air with both hands and catch it when it comes back down. Make the two sides of your body move exactly the same way.
2. Throw and catch the beanbag with both hands. Make the beanbag just touch the ceiling.

Level 2:
1. Throw and catch the beanbag with both hands. Throw the beanbag up and try to make it come 1 foot from the ceiling, then 2 feet from the ceiling, and then 3 feet from the ceiling. Continue this sequence.
2. Throw and catch the beanbag with the right hand and follow the motion of the beanbag with your hands.

Level 3:
1. Throw and catch the beanbag with your right hand. Make the beanbag just touch the ceiling.
2. Throw and catch the beanbag with your left hand. Make the beanbag come as close to the ceiling as you possibly can without touching the ceiling.
3. Throw and catch the beanbag with your right hand. Make the beanbag come to within 1 foot of the ceiling. The next time make it come within 2 feet of the ceiling. The next time make it come within 3 feet of the ceiling.

Level 4:
1. Throw and catch the beanbag with both hands. Make the beanbag come as close to the ceiling as possible when you throw it up and let it get as close to the floor as possible before you catch it.
2. Throw the beanbag up with your right hand. Make the beanbag come as close to the ceiling as possible when you throw it up and let it get as close to the floor as possible before you catch it. Catch it with your right hand.
3. Invent your own way to throw and catch the beanbag.

Level 5:
1. Throw the beanbag up with both hands and catch it on the back of your right hand when it comes back down.
2. Throw the beanbag up with both hands and catch it on the back of your left hand when it comes back down.
3. Put the beanbag on the back of both hands. Throw the beanbag up in the air and catch it.
4. Throw the beanbag in the air and when it reaches its trajectory, close your eyes. Try to catch the beanbag with your eyes closed.

Form GM-16 (continued)
BEANBAG ACTIVITIES

5. Throw and catch two beanbags simultaneously. Throw and catch the lightest beanbag with your right hand and the heaviest beanbag with your left hand.

6. Throw and catch two beanbags simultaneously. Throw and catch the heaviest one with your left hand and the lightest one with your right hand. Throw them as high up in the air as you can and keep them under control. Try to throw them up and just touch the ceiling. Try to make both of them go up the same distance when you throw them.

7. Throw the two beanbags in the air and clap a rhythm pattern before catching the bags.

Form GM-17
BALANCE BOARD ON HANDS AND KNEES

Purpose: Gross motor, vestibular.

Materials: Marsden ball, balance board, metronome, fixation chart.

Method: Have the child get on his hands and knees on the balance board. Make sure he keeps his head up and looks straight ahead.

Level 1: Child is to keep his balance on the board as he looks straight ahead. See how long he can keep his balance.

Level 2: Have him move his head back and forth (right to left) as he keeps his balance. Hold your thumbs about 24 inches apart and directly in front of him. Have him move his eyes quickly from thumb to thumb.

Level 3:
1. Do four corner fixations. Have the child stare straight ahead. At the beat of the metronome, he moves his eyes quickly to the top right corner of the wall, then the bottom right corner, then the bottom left corner and then the top left corner. He moves his eyes each time the metronome beats. He is not to move his head, only his eyes.
2. Have him track the Marsden ball in a left to right direction. Have the ball hung so that it is at his eye level. He moves his eyes only, not his head.
3. Swing the ball around his head in a circular fashion and see if he can keep his head and eyes on it without losing his balance.

Levels 4 and 5: Put a number fixation chart directly in front of him on the wall. As he keeps his balance, he is to call out the numbers as fast as he can. You can go in the horizontal or vertical direction. He moves his eyes only, not his head.

Fixation Chart

1	9	2	1	3	5	4	7
3	8	3	7	6	3	2	5
4	6	5	1	8	6	1	3
5	3	7	3	2	9	4	6
6	4	8	4	1	7	8	2
7	2	9	5	9	3	9	4
8	9	2	7	5	1	6	3
9	5	1	6	3	2	7	4
8	3	5	8	2	1	3	7
5	1	6	7	8	2	4	3

Form GM-18
VMC Bat While Balancing

Purpose: Gross motor, vestibular, laterality.

Materials: VMC bat, Marsden ball, balance disc. The VMC bat is a dowel rod about 3 feet in length and 1 inch in diameter. It is divided into various colored sections.

Methods: He does these activities while he is standing on the balance disc or the end of the walking rail.

Level 1: Have the child hit the ball by pushing the bat at it. See how long he can do it without missing the ball.

Level 2: You call out various colors on the bat and have him hit the ball with that color. He always hits the ball by pushing the bat (not like a baseball bat).

Levels 3 to 5:
1. Call out a side and color and have the child hit the ball with that color, for example, "right red" or "left blue".
2. Have him hit various colors in sequence. For example, "right red", "left blue", and "right green". Have him hit it a number of times with one color and another number of times with another color. For example, ten times with the "right red" and three times with the "left blue".

Form GM-19
TAPE WALKING

Purpose: Gross motor, vestibular.

Materials: Masking tape.

Method: Put an 8-foot long strip of fairly wide masking tape on the floor. The child is to do the following activities walking in a heel to toe manner on the tape. He is to walk so that the heel of one foot touches the toes of the other. He is not to have his shoes on and should always have good posture and keep his head and eyes straight ahead.

Level 1: Tell the child to do the following.
1. Walk forward on the tape. (Child keeps his eyes on a target in front of him.)
2. Walk forward on the tape and carry a weight in your left hand.
3. Walk forward on the tape and carry a weight in your right hand.
4. Walk forward on the tape and change the weight from hand to hand.
5. Walk backward on the tape.
6. Walk backward on the tape and carry a weight in your left hand.
7. Invent your own way to cross the tape.

Level 2: Tell the child to do the following.
1. Walk backward on the tape and change the weight from hand to hand.
2. Walk forward on the tape with a book balanced on your head.
3. Walk backward on the tape with a book balanced on your head.
4. Walk on the tape with a book balanced on your head and carry a weight.
5. Walk on the tape and throw a beanbag at a target on command.
6. Walk on the tape and catch a beanbag and throw it back.
7. Walk on the tape and bounce a ball as you walk.
8. Walk sideways on the tape and lead with your right foot.
9. Walk sideways on the tape and lead with your left foot.
10. Walk sideways on the tape and carry a weight in one of your hands.
11. Walk sideways on the tape and change a weight from hand to hand.
12. Walk sideways on the tape with a book balanced on your head and carry a weight in your hand.
13. Walk sideways on the tape with a weight in your hand. In the middle of the tape, turn around and walk backward to the end.
14. Walk on the tape with your arms extended to the sides, then to the front, back both to one side, and then both to the other side.
15. Walk on the tape with your arms extended in front, back to opposite sides, then both to one side, and both to the other side.
16. Walk forward with your left foot always in front of the right.
17. Walk forward with your right foot always in front of the left.
18. Walk backward with your right foot always in front of the left.
19. Walk backward with your left foot always in front of the right.
20. Invent five activities.

Form GM-20
WALKING RAIL/BALANCE BEAM

Purpose: Gross motor, vestibular.

Materials: Walking rail, various objects to carry: book, yardstick, playground ball, and beanbag. You will need an 8-foot long, 2 inch x 4 inch board that has been sanded so there are no rough places. You will need three 1-foot long 4 inch x 4 inch blocks of wood. Lay the 2 inch x 4 inch board on the blocks of wood to make the walking rail.

Method: Tell the child to do the following activities. Always make sure he has good posture with his head up and eyes looking straight ahead. When he walks on the rail, have him walk in a heel to toe manner. His heel should touch his toe on each step. Always have the child take his shoes off and walk on the rail in his socks or bare feet.

Note: If Level 1 of this activity is too difficult for the child, and he has an extremely difficult time balancing on the board, switch to activities in GM-19.

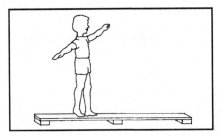

Level 1: Tell the child to do the following.
1. Walk forward across the board. Keep your eyes on a target in front of you.
2. Walk forward across the board and carry a weight in your left hand.
3. Walk forward across the board and carry the weight in your right hand.
4. Walk forward across the board and change the weight from hand to hand.

Level 2: Tell the child to do the following.
1. Walk backward across the board.
2. Walk backward across the board and carry a weight in your left hand.
3. Invent your own way to cross the board.
4. Walk backward across the board and change the weight from hand to hand.
5. Walk forward across the board with a book balanced on your head.
6. Walk backward across the board with a book balanced on your head.
7. Walk forward across the board with a book balanced on your head and carry a weight.
8. Walk across the board and throw a beanbag at a target on command.
9. Walk forward across the board and catch a beanbag and throw it back.
10. Walk across the board with your arms extended to the sides; then to the front, back, both to one side, then both to the other side.
11. Walk across the board with your arms extended in front, back to opposite sides, and then both to one side, then both to the other side.
12. Walk backward with your left foot always in front of the right.
13. Walk backward with your right foot always in front of the left.
14. Walk backward with your left foot always in front of the right.
15. Invent five activities.

Form GM-20 (continued)
WALKING RAIL/BALANCE BEAM

Level 3: Tell the child to do the following.
1. Walk forward and pick up a book from the center of the beam.
2. Walk backward and pick up a book from the center of the beam.
3. Have someone hold a yardstick 12 inches over the center of the beam. Walk to the center and step over the yardstick.
4. Increase the height of the step as necessary to clear the yardstick.
5. Walk across the beam in various ways. Have someone stand at the end of the board with a target. Watch the target as you move across the beam.
6. Invent seven ways to cross the board that have not been covered.
7. Teacher or parent holds a yardstick at a height of 3 feet. Walk forward and pass under the yardstick.
8. Go under and over the yardstick. Teacher varies the position of the yardstick both in height and in position relative to the length of the beam.
9. Walk the beam forward with your arms out, palms down with a book on the back of each hand.
10. Invent five ways to cross the board using the books balanced on your hands.
11. Invent three new ways to cross the board.
12. Go to the center of the board. Catch a beanbag and throw it back to the teacher or parent or at a target. Move to various positions on the board and repeat throwing the beanbag. Teacher or parent remains in one place.
13. Go to the center of the board. Teacher or parent goes to the end of the beam to face you. Move arms and legs in various positions exactly as teacher or parent does. (If child's position is not correct, call his attention to the fact.)
14. Teacher or parent places a bucket at the end of the beam and throws you a beanbag. Walk towards the bucket, catch the beanbag, and try to throw the beanbag into the bucket without looking at it.
15. Place a book at the middle of the beam. Walk the beam sideways and pick up the book, turn around and walk to the end of the beam.
16. Invent seven ways to cross the beam using all three of the items: the yardstick, the book, and the beanbag.
17. Teacher or parent holds the yardstick at various heights above the beam. Put your hands on your hips and walk backward under the yardstick.
18. With your arms held sideways, walk to the middle of the beam, turn around, and walk backward.
19. Walk forward with your hands on hips.
20. Walk backward with your hands on hips.
21. Place book at center of beam. Walk to center, place the book on the top of your head, and then continue to the end of beam.

Level 4: Tell the child to do the following.
1. Walk backward and pass under yardstick held by the teacher or parent.
2. Walk the beam backward with your hands clasped behind your body.
3. Walk the beam forward, arms held sideways, palms up, with a book on the palm of each hand.
4. Walk the beam backward, arms held sideways, palms up, with a book on the palm of each hand.
5. Walk the beam sideways, right, weight on balls of feet.
6. Walk the beam sideways, left, weight on balls of feet.
7. Clasp arms in read and walk across the board.

Form GM-20 (continued)
WALKING RAIL/BALANCE BEAM

8. Invent seven different ways to cross the board with arms in various positions.
9. Invent seven different ways to cross the board with one arm held in various positions.
10. Walk to the center of the board, stand on your left foot and balance.
11. Devise five activities to do with your eyes closed.
12. Walk to the middle of the beam. Balance on one foot then turn around on that foot and walk backward to the end of the beam.
13. Walk to the middle of the beam, left sideways, turn around and walk to the end of the beam, right sideways.
14. With your arms clasped behind your body, walk forward to the middle, turn around once, walk backward the remaining distance.

Level 5: Tell the child to do the following.
1. Stand on beam, one foot in front of the other, keep your eyes closed, and maintain your balance as long as possible. Record number of seconds.
2. Stand on your right foot, eyes closed, and maintain your balance as long as possible. Record number of seconds.
3. Stand on your left foot, eyes closed, and maintain your balance as long as possible. Record number of seconds.
4. Walk beam sideways, left eye closed.

Form GM-21
TRAMPOLINE

Purpose: Gross motor, vestibular.

Materials: Trampoline (a small trampoline is adequate), metronome, fixation chart (see Form GM-17).

Method: Have the child do the following on the trampoline.

Level 1: Have the child jump on the trampoline, trying to stay in one place. You are looking for good form with both of his feet touching the trampoline at the same time.

Level 2:
1. While the child is jumping, have him catch a beanbag and throw it back to you.
2. While the child is jumping, have him hold a weight in one hand (a weight can be any small object, for example, a flashlight).
3. Same as # 2, but have him swing the weighted hands through various motions as he jumps on the trampoline.
4. As the child jumps, he is to alternate back and forth once on each foot.
5. Have him jump on the left foot twice, the right foot once. Vary this activity. For example, right foot twice, left foot three times.

Level 3:
1. Have the child jump and clap his hands to various rhythmic combinations.
2. Have him jump and call out the letters in a left to right sequence on the fixation chart. Add the metronome and have him call out a letter to each beat of the metronome.
3. Have the child hop and do jumping jacks. He is to keep his arms and legs working together in a synchronized manner.
4. Have him hold a beanbag in each hand and do jumping jacks.
5. Have him do jumping jacks and switch the beanbag from hand to hand when his hands are in the overhead position.
6. As the child is doing jumping jacks, on command have him drop both of his arms without disturbing the total pattern.
7. As the child is doing jumping jacks, on command have him drop just his left or right arm.

Levels 4 and 5:
1. As the child is doing jumping jacks, on command he is to drop his right arm for two jumps, and bring it back for two jumps. Then he is to drop his left arm for two jumps and bring it back for two jumps.
2. Have him jump in a cross pattern. He is to move his right arm and his left leg forward as he moves his left arm and right leg back.

Form GM-22
Jump Rope Activities

Purpose: Gross motor.

Materials: 7 foot jump rope, metronome.

Method: The child should do all these activities with relaxed knees, a straight but not stiff back, and his head held up. If the child cannot swing the rope himself and jump at the same time, tie one end to a chair and swing the other end for him.

Level 1: Do these activities with the rope laying on the floor.
1. With the rope laying in a straight line, have the child place a foot on either side of the rope and jump to the opposite end forward and return to the starting end with backward jumps.
2. With the rope in a circle, jump with feet together in and out of the circle.
3. With the rope in a circle, place one foot on the inside and the other on the outside of the circle. Jump around the circle to the starting place.

Level 2: One end of the rope is in each hand.
1. Swing the rope back and forth under the body and jump with feet together each time it goes under the body.
2. Same as #1, but use only the right foot.
3. Same as #1, but use only the left foot.
4. Swing the rope over the head and under the body, jumping each time it goes under the body. Jump with both feet at the same time.

Levels 3 to 5: One end of the rope is in each hand.
1. Swing the rope over the head and under the body, jumping each time it goes under the body. Jump with both feet at the same time. Do one jump for each beat of the metronome. Set the metronome at a very slow cadence for this activity and then work up to faster speed.
2. Same as #1, but alternate feet for each beat.

Form GM-23
RHYTHM

Purpose: Cerebellum activation.

Materials: Metronome.

Method: The child is to reproduce the rhythm pattern. Sit opposite the child at a table.

Level 1: Beat out a constant rhythm pattern with one of your hands. Have the child look at you and do the same. Don't do more than a two beat rhythm. For example: da-dit, da-dit, da-dit.

Level 2:
1. Use a two beat rhythm and beat out a rhythm pattern with one of your hands. Have him look at you and do the same.
2. Same as #1, but have the child close his eyes and try to match your rhythm pattern.
3. Same as #1 and #2, but use a three beat rhythm. For example: da-dit-dit, da-dit-dit.
4. Beat out a constant rhythm pattern alternating between hands. The child watches you and repeats the rhythm with his hands. For example: R-L-R-L.
5. Do double alterations. For example: R-R-L-L-R-R.
6. Do three alterations. For example: RRR-LLL.
7. Do irregular rhythm. For example: RR-L RR-L. Vary these patterns.

Level 3: Beat out a constant rhythm with your hands on the table. Child has his eyes closed. Start with double alterations, for example, R-R-L-L-R-R, then three alterations R-R-R-L-L-L, and finally irregular rhythm R-R-R-L-L-R-R. The child then copies your rhythm.

Level 4:
1. This is done with a metronome. The child is to touch his thumb to one of his fingers on the same hand at the beat of the metronome. Assign numbers to the fingers. Have him touch the sequence you want to the beat of the metronome. For example: 2, 3, 4 or 2, 4, 5.

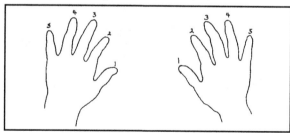

2. Use both hands. For example: 3, 2, 4 on the right and 3, 2, 4 on the left.

Level 5:
1. This is done with a metronome, with his eyes closed. The child is to touch his thumb to one of his fingers at the beat of the metronome. Assign numbers to his fingers. Have him touch the sequence you want. For example: 2, 3, 4, 5 or 2, 4, 5.
2. With his eyes closed, alternate hands. For example: 2, 4, 5 right, 2, 5 left.
3. Do #1 and 2 again, but with his eyes open, he is to touch the thumb of one hand to the fingers of the other.

Form GM-24
RHYTHM-2

Purpose: Cerebellum stimulation.

Materials: For Levels 3 to 5, cards with dots drawn on them. Below is an example of the cards.

Method: The child will follow the therapist's instruction. When the cards are used, dots close together require a fast beat, far apart is a slow beat, and the space in between is a pause. For example:

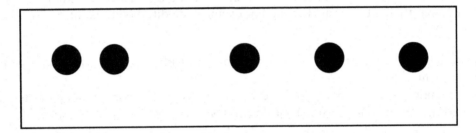

This is two fast, pause, three slow.

Level 1:
1. Tell the child to take a pencil and tap the same pattern as you do.
2. Tell the child to tap the pencil very fast, then very slowly. Tell him to continue until you tell him to stop.

Level 2: You tap out a pattern using the pencil or your feet and hands and the child does the same thing.

Level 3: Now use the dot cards that you have made in advance. Show him one card. Let him look at it, and while he is still looking at it, clap the pattern on the card.

Levels 4 and 5:
1. Same as Level 3, but take the card away and have him clap from memory.
2. You clap a pattern and then show the child several cards. He is to point to the card that has the pattern you clapped.

Form GM-25
FINGER TO THUMB

Purpose: Cerebellum stimulation and eye-hand coordination.

Materials: Metronome.

Method: At the beat of the metronome, the child will touch the tips of the fingers of one hand with the thumb of the other hand. The child should start either standing or seated.

Level 1: Set the metronome at a low level. At each beat, have the child touch any finger on his left hand with the thumb of his right hand. If the child is left-handed, use his left hand and touch tips of his right hand.

Level 2: At the beat of the metronome, the child will touch the fingers of one hand with the thumb of the other hand in the sequence from the thumb to the little finger. Then go back in the reverse sequence of little finger to thumb.

Level 3:
1. Same as Level 2, but then switch hands after completion with one hand.
2. Use other fingers in place of the thumb, and speed up the metronome.

Levels 4 and 5: Same as Level 3 but vary the activities. Some examples are:
1. Touch every other finger.
2. Touch the tip of the nose and alternate between the nose and the fingers. For example: thumb of one hand to thumb of the other hand, then the thumb to the tip of the nose, then the thumb to the index finger, etc.

Form GM-26
DUAL-TASK

Purpose: Cerebellum and vestibular stimulation.

Materials: Walking rail or balance disc, marking board.

Method: The idea of this exercise is to stimulate several areas simultaneously. Use as many auditory, balance, and visual aids as possible. The child will stand in a heel to toe manner on the walking rail or feet together on the disc. He is to keep his balance as he does these activities.

Levels 3 to 5:
1. Have the child solve simple math problems that you have written on the board.
2. Play tic-tac-toe on the board.
3. He tells you where to place his X. In one grid, draw an X. Let him see it for a few seconds and then stand in front of it. Do spatial memory games. You draw two grids of squares. He is to tell you in which square in his grid to put the X to match yours. Build up to several Xs to make it difficult.
4. Name a word and have him say a word that rhymes with it.
5. Say words and have him repeat them with a syllable missing. For example, say "cowboy" without the "cow".
6. Use the letter chart and have him call the letters out in a row as fast as he can.
7. Hold a book in front of him, and have him read it aloud to you.
8. Have him name as many words as he can that start with F. Pick other letters.
9. Make up as many activities as you can.

Form GM-27
RHYME/SOUND CATEGORIZATION

Purpose: To train cerebellum functions.

Materials: Walking rail.

Method: As the child is slowly walking on the walking rail, ask him the following questions without his losing his balance.

Level 3: These are examples of the types of questions for Level 3.
1. "Name a word that rhymes with *cat*."
2. "Does *cat* rhyme with *map?*"
3. "Make up words that rhyme."

Level 4: Do Level 3 plus the following types of questions.
1. "Do *map* and *man* start with the same sound?"
2. "Make up words that start with the same sound."

Level 5: Do Levels 3 and 4 plus the following types of questions. Tell the child a category. Have him think of words that rhyme with something in that category. Both words don't have to be from the same category. For example: You say "farming", and he says "cow - plow". You say "sports" and he says "ball - hall".

Form GM-28
MENTAL ROTATIONS

Purpose: Cerebellum activation for visual spatial abilities.

Materials: Small colored blocks.

Method: The child is to follow your instruction and design his blocks the way you ask him.

Level 3: Tell the child, "I want you to look at the blocks I have put on the table, and show me with your blocks what it would look like backwards" (or reversed, whichever he understands). For example:

R   R   B   Y   G

This reversed would be:

G   Y   B   R   R

Make up various designs for him to show you what they would look like if they were backwards or reversed.

R   R
B   B
Y   Y
G   R   B   Y   Y   B   R   G

Levels 4 and 5:
Now ask the child what your blocks would look like if they were rotated (turned). For example, what would these blocks look like if they were rotated clockwise 90 degrees?

R   G   Y   R   R
R   ⟶   B
Y   R
G   B   R   Y

If you keep rotating it clockwise, what would it look like?

Y   R   B   G   Y
               Y   ⟶   R
               R   B
               R   R   R   Y   G

Make up various designs. For example:

R   G   Y
B
Y
R   R   G   B

Form GM-29
VISUAL IMAGERY

Purpose: Activation of brain areas associated with motor activities.

Materials: Metronome.

Method: Everyone starts at Level 1. Have the child stand up and close his eyes (if he has difficulty with this, have him do it seated). Always have him take a few deep breaths before you start the activity.

Level 1:
1. Do this level seated. Ask him to pretend he sees himself seated at the table. Ask him if he sees something else on the table. Get him to verbalize what he is pretending to see.
2. Tell him not to really move his hand off of the table, but pretend he sees himself doing it. Ask questions. For example, which hand did he move? Touch his hand and ask: "Is this the hand?"
3. Ask him to pretend to move the other hands off of the table so that he sees himself with both hands off of the table.
4. Now have him pretend to move both hands back on the table.

Level 2:
1. Do this level seated. Ask him to pretend he is holding both of his hands straight up in the air. Each time you say "one", he is to pretend to move one of his hands back to the table with the other hand still in the air. When you say "two", he moves the other hand that is still in the air back to the table and moves the other hand that was on the table back into the air.
2. Now each time you clap, he moves his hands, one on top of the table and the other in the air. He switches each time you clap.

Level 3:
1. The child is standing with his eyes closed. He now pretends that he does not see himself as if he is looking at himself from a distance but sees himself as if he is actually performing the task. He pretends that he is looking through his own eyes.
2. Have him pretend his is bouncing a ball with his right hand. Each time, it hits the floor, he says "hit".
3. Have him bounce but switch hands.
4. Have him pretend he is throwing it against the wall and catching it. When it hits the wall, he says "hit". When he catches it, he says "catch".

Level 4:
1. Same as Level 3. He pretends he is looking through his eyes. The child is standing with his eyes closed.
2. Have him pretend he is bouncing the ball off of the wall. Each time he hears the metronome, have him throw the ball and catch it. Have him switch hands.
3. He pretends his arms are at his side. Each time he hears the metronome, he pretends to clap his hands over his head.

Level 5:
1. Same as Levels 3 and 4. He pretends he is looking through his eyes. The child is standing with his eyes closed.
2. Have him pretend he is doing jumping jacks. At each beat of the metronome, he does one jumping jack.
3. Make up different activities.

Chapter Six

VISUAL MOTOR PERCEPTION

"Neither can there be a perception taking place without activity which involves motor elements". (Piaget, 1948)

Visual motor perception is the ability to copy geometric shapes, letters, or drawings in a proper spatial manner. It involves using spatial relationships, memory, fine motor development, visual perception, visuospatial encoding, motor planning, sequencing, and cognition (pertaining to mental processes and reasoning). Handwriting is a fine motor skill but does not require the same degree of motor planning, cognition, or perceptual development as visual-motor perception. While visual motor skills would involve reaching, grasping, and visual guidance of hand and arm movement, visual motor perception involves the ability to reproduce shapes and letters properly. Most experts agree that a child has to reach a certain degree of maturity in visual motor perception before he is able to learn reading, writing, and the comprehension of number concepts (Kopptiz, 1963). For this reason, visual motor perception is critical for school achievement because it is so closely related to language ability and other functions associated with young children, such as memory, visual perception, motor coordination, temporal and spatial concepts, and organization (Kopptiz, 1963).

Form-copy tests are excellent indicators of a child's future school performance. If I had to choose only one test to give a child to determine his school readiness, it would undoubtedly be the form-copy test. This, in conjunction with speed in symbol naming (letters, numerals), has generally been among the strongest predictors of reading achievement (Mati-Zissi, 2001). Correlations between form-copy tests and readiness tests in kindergarten often range from .50 to .70. Similarly, correlations between form copying and early reading achievement range between .40 and .60 (.00 is no relationship to 1.00, which is perfect relationship) (Beery, 1982).

The deficiencies children experience in drawing seem to be attributable to problems in visuospatial perception, planning, and short-term memory. There seems to be a high positive correlation between reading accuracy in decoding in grade three and early drawing depiction in preschoolers. The highest positive correlations appear in spatial relationships, direction orientation programming and sequencing, as well as the application of rules that accompany all of the above. These early sequencing difficulties may account for decoding deficiencies experienced later. Also worth mentioning is the high positive correlation that appears between the drawing factors and storing and recalling abilities of short-term phonological working memory (Mati-Zissi, 2001).

Before we get into a more detailed description of children's drawings and the motor planning involved, we need to discuss the development of children's spatial relations and perceptual space.

The development of the perception of spatial relations is divided into three periods. The first period is up to 5 months of age and is divided into five spatial relationships:

1. The most elementary spatial relationship is *proximity*, or the nearness of objects.

2. The second spatial relationship is *separation*, as in one object being separated from another.

3. The third relationship is *succession*. For example, when two neighboring though separate elements are arranged one before another (the relation of order or spatial succession), such as the sight of a door opening and a figure appearing.

4. The fourth spatial relationship is *enclosure*. An example would be an object in a box.

5. The fifth spatial relationship is *continuity*, or the quality of being continuous. For example, the case of unbroken lines on a surface.

The second period of spatial relations is from 5 months to 12 months. This period evolves as a result of sensorimotor development. It is marked by the coordination of vision and the child's ability to distinguish his own movements from an object's. Movements and tactile exploration all play a fundamental part in this development. This period starts the development of constancies of shape and size, such as perceiving the true dimensions of an object seen from a distance (at 8 to 10 months). At this stage, the child is also able to reverse a feeding bottle that is presented to him the wrong way (8 to 9 months).

The third period begins at 12 months. Whereas the achievements of the second period are essentially relative to the shape and dimensions of objects, those of the third period consist in bringing out the relationships of objects to each other. This is the stage where the first attempts to draw are initiated due to the start of the mental image. It is worth noting that despite their differences and the time lag that separates them, both perceptual and representational construction to some extent possess a factor in common. This common factor is *motor activity* (Piaget, 1948).

Once the concepts of spatial relations has been mastered, the child is now capable of understanding perceptual space, both in recognition and of drawing. The concept of perceptual space is organized in three successive stages.

1. Up to 4 years: The only shapes that are recognized or drawn are closed, rounded shapes that are based on simple topological relations such as openness, closure, proximity, and separation.

2. 4 years to 7 years: In this stage, we encounter the

beginning of recognition or drawing of Euclidean shapes (e. g., a diamond), based on the distinction between straight and curved lines, angles of different sizes, parallels, and especially on relations between equal or unequal sides of a figure.

3. 7 years to 8 years: In this stage, one finds the child capable of being able to use a point of reference. For example, when a child draws a six-pointed star, he will use the center as a reference point to draw each arm of the star. Also at this stage, the child can draw an object by deriving a mental image of it by using tactile and kinesthetic information (Piaget, 1948).

In order to appreciate the importance of children's drawings and their relation to learning disabilities, I need to stress that many of the same factors that are needed to properly reproduce a drawing are also needed in such school subjects as reading and spelling. These include: short-term memory, visual perception, visuospatial encoding, planning, sequencing, perception of shape, position, and spatial orientation (Mati-Zissi, 1998).

Recent research findings have indicated that the problems of children with special learning difficulties were attributed to deficits in the visual-analysis system and visual-input lexicon (Ellis, 1995). The visual-analysis system, a nonlexical system, recognizes and indicates the position of the letter symbols inside the word. This system stores the visual information in short-term memory to analyze it in its graphemic constituents and eventually passes it on to a long-term memory of graphemes known as the visual-input lexicon. Perception of shape, form, and position of symbols is, therefore, a significant component of the reading mechanism. Equally important for the reading process is the grapheme-phoneme correspondence that is the conversion of words into syllable codes. A similar system of visual analysis occurs in the drawing process. The visual analysis system analyzes those drawing symbols, such as spots, lines, circles, and squares, which form the drawing units. The combination of these units leads to the production of drawings (Mati-Zissi, 2001). A necessary prerequisite for correct depiction of objects is perception of shape, spatial orientation, and position. Drawing performance is also facilitated by recalling familiar picture representations stored in memory. Children with learning difficulties show deficient drawing skills, and therefore, difficult drawing strategies because their drawing mechanisms for correct depiction appear to be malfunctioning (Mati-Zissi, 2001).

It is important to remember that children's drawings involve more than eye-hand coordination. Drawing is a fine motor skill that involves perception and memory. I have often seen children with normal eye-hand coordination who have poor visual motor perceptual skills. Visual motor perceptual skills must be developed. You can't

expect to have a 4-year-old draw a vertical diamond. To stress the point that children's drawings are much more than just fine motor skills, research has shown that it is just as difficult for a child to make a square with four matchsticks as it is to draw it. A child cannot form a square or a triangle with matchsticks any earlier than he can draw them (Piaget, 1948). Therefore, we may assume that the problem is not one that depends upon mere motor ability, but rather in the method of composition itself.

A child's first attempts at drawing occur between 18 months and 2 years. These are scribbles and are not intended to represent anything. The child is just moving his arm in a rhythmic motion (Thomas, 1990). From 2½ years, children see their drawings as representations of something (Thomas, 1990). By 4, attribution of meaning is found in two-thirds of the drawings (Piaget, 1948). A child should be able to draw a square at 4 years, a triangle from 4.6 to 5.6 years, and a vertical diamond at age 6. It takes 2 years of development for a child to progress from drawing a square to a diamond.

It has been noticed that children often use similar drawing methods. A preference for starting at the top and at the left seems to appear at an age before children learn to read or write, and it persists regardless of the direction of the script they learn to use (English, Arabic, Hebrew and so forth) (Thomas, 1990). The Grammar of Action Rule states that American children use similar principles in copying geometric shapes. These include:

1. Start at the topmost point.
2. Start at the left most point.
3. With the vertical line, start at the top and come down the left oblique when the figure has an apex.
4. Draw all horizontal lines left to right.
5. Draw all vertical lines top to bottom.
6. Threading (joined lines) (Wann, 1991).

It has also been noticed that the velocity of a movement is proportionally tied to its linear extension (or trajectory's length) so that the execution time is maintained. Thus, the circle of a large diameter is drawn in the same amount of time as is a smaller diameter (Isochrery Principle) (Wann, 1991). It has been discovered that children may draw vertical and horizontal lines most accurately due to the abundance of vertical and horizontal lines in our environment. Recognition and discrimination also may be influenced by the surroundings, e.g., the paper they are drawing on (picture frame clues). Square and rectangle picture frame clues may aid in the discrimination of horizontal and vertical lines (Broderick, 1987).

The question we have to ask is why does it take 2 years of development for a child to go from drawing a square to a vertical diamond? We know the answer is more complex than just developing eye-hand coordination. In fact, fine motor ability cannot be the cause for greater efficiency in copying squares versus diamonds. A child at age 5 can trace over the lines of a diamond as accurately as a square. The implications are that planning of action (motor planning) and/or processing feedback information could be responsible for the differential difficulty in copying the two figures (Broderick, 1987; Mati-Zissi, 1998). The drawing of a shape, whether simple or complex, involves a number of decisions. These include positioning, sequencing, and motor planning. A child of 4 does not have the skills that are needed to draw oblique lines and angles that are required for a vertical diamond. When attempting to copy figures from models, the first task requirement is visual recognition and/or discrimination of the presented model figures. Visual recognition and discrimination are followed by generating a plan of action. Before the start of a movement, a movement plan has to be ready. The plan of action relevant to the copying task includes such factors as selection of the starting point, direction and speed of movement, and definition of the force exerted on the drawing implement. Activation of the specific motor units, selection of appropriate number of motor units, and the temporal sequencing of their activation are the motor programming parameters. These parameters relate to the direction, extent of force, and speed of the ensuing movement. During the execution of the movement, visual and kinesthetic feedback is generated. With the aid of feedback, errors in movement are detected, and corrective programming is initiated (Broderick, 1987). Motor planning is an integral part of the perceptual motor system and is not a conscious process. The motor plan is formulated according to information stored in memory about the movement. The effectiveness of the motor plan depends on efficient processing and storage of the relevant kinesthetic information. This is why training is essential for proper visual motor perceptual skills.

I mentioned earlier that many of the factors that are required to complete a visual motor perceptual task are the same ones that are involved in such school activities as reading. It is, therefore, not surprising that many dyslexic children have poor visual motor perceptual skills. It appears that dyslexics have problems in spatial orientation and lack proper planning of the actions required of the drawing task (Mati-Zissi, 1998). It also appears that the perception of the position, the limits and distances between the drawn parts of pictures, the orientation of the various figures, their sequence and the conception itself of each form all appear to develop in dyslexic children in the same peculiar manner they develop in reading and writing (Mati-Zissi, 1998). The writing performance of dyslexic individuals most often reflects disturbances in graphomotor and spatial coordination. Pencils are often awkwardly and tightly held. Their writing is slowly and meticulously executed in an attempt to compensate for underlying disorganizing tendencies that are analogous to those scrambling the dyslexic reading process. Letters and words are often poorly formed, spaced, and directed, and sentences tend to drift off the horizontal (Levinson, 1980). Other characteristics of dyslexics include omission of words or letters, lack of rhythm, large width or larger than average letter size, and heavier than normal pressure, which is often irregular (Wann, 1991). However, it should be stressed that not all dyslexics have poor visual motor perceptual skills, nor should it be assumed just because a child has sloppy or disorganized drawing and writing skills, that he is dyslexic. Just as dyslexia represents the lower 2 to 4% of the reading population, dysgraphia represents the lower end of the writing population. *Dysgraphia* is a writing disorder evidenced in children of at least average intelligence and has no distinct neurological cause. It is a written-language disorder that concerns mechanical writing skills and is unrelated to other learning disabilities such as reading, spelling, or math (Hamstra-Bletz, 1990). The problems of dysgraphic writers appear to relate to a lack of fine motor control in the execution of these programs. It is likely that something goes wrong in choosing movement parameters, which results in errors in the direction and/or relative size of the movement components (Hamstra-Bletz, 1990). There does not appear to be a higher percentage of dysgraphics among left handers than among right handers (Maeland, 1992), and dysgraphic and nondysgraphic writers do not differ in speed (Hamstra-Bletz, 1990). It has been suggested that dysgraphia for letters may represent a specific type of motor memory deficit dissociable from copying skills and the ability to draw letter-like forms (Kapur, 1983).

According to the most recent theories on dysgraphia, it is characterized by two different groups of deficits. The first group, neglect-related features, is represented by the tendency to write on the right hand side of the page and by difficulty maintaining horizontal lines. Omissions and repetitions of strokes and letters form the second group of dysgraphic deficits (Strauss, 1979). The following are symptoms often associated with dysgraphia:

1. Odd wrist, body, or paper positions.
2. Excessive erasures, especially due to faulty letter form.
3. Inconsistent letter formations and slant.
4. Irregular letter sizes and shapes.
5. Unfinished cursive letters.
6. Cramped fingers on the writing tool.
7. Inappropriate mixture of upper and lower case letters.

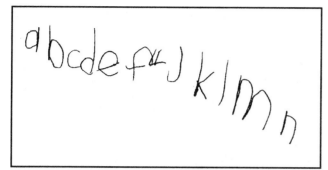

Figure 6-1. Poor organization on page.

8. Mixture of printed and cursive letters.
9. Misuse of line and margin .
10. Poor organization on page (Figure 6-1).
11. Inefficient speed in copying.
12. Decreased or increased speed in writing.
13. General illegibility.
14. Inattentiveness about details when writing.

There are several factors that exacerbate motor memory problems. The first two factors always indicate dysgraphia and the last two factors by themselves rarely indicate dysgraphia.

1. Weak kinesthetic memory so that an accurate pattern is not stored.
2. Poor ability to express written ideas with clarity and in sequence, especially when the student is more efficient when verbally expressing clear, sequential ideas.
3. Generalized memory or sequencing weakness.
4. Weak or inconsistent ability to recall visual and motor movement sequences.
5. Inexperience due to lack of practice involving consistent repetition of the pattern.
6. Lack of experience due to attentional problems (Richards, 1999).

Dysgraphia is a problem that is not due to attentional problems or lack of practice. Handwriting that is sloppy and disorganized deteriorates over the years and becomes practically illegible because of changes in structural performance. Dysgraphic handwriting shows poor structural performance from the beginning. The differences between dysgraphic and nondysgraphic handwriting are the largest in grade two (Hamstra-Bletz, 1990). Keep in mind that just as dyslexic readers are poor readers from the beginning, dysgraphic writers are poor writers from the beginning. Dysgraphia is not the result of poor instruction or lack of training (Van Galen, 1993).

Poor handwriting is one of the most frequent reasons that school aged children are referred to occupational therapy (Fisher, 1991). Ten to 20% of primary school children have dysfunctional handwriting, and among those 66% are boys (Karlsdottir, 1996). Handwriting goes through several stages, with the mastery of most forms and some manuscript letters in preschool and kindergarten to mastery of upper and lower case manuscript in grades one to the beginning of two. In grades two to four, cursive writing is introduced (Richards, 1999). There is initially fast improvement in handwriting in first and second grades; however, the quality of handwriting tends to stagnate after third grade (Karlsdottir, 2002). Initially, the size of handwriting becomes smaller over time (especially boys), the word and letter alignment improves, the writing trace becomes steadier, and the lines are smooth. Girls are ahead of boys in development. Later on, when formal instruction in handwriting has stopped, the handwriting changes and some deterioration of form starts to develop (Hamstra-Bletz, 1990). From fourth grade on, children start to use easier movement patterns that require less effort. In addition, in higher grades, the script becomes larger, joins between letters are often omitted, and the letters are placed very closely together (Hamstra-Bletz, 1990).

It appears that most improvements in handwriting occur over the first three grades. In fact, children with functional handwriting at the end of first grade don't make any significant improvements in their handwriting during the higher grades. Good handwriters reach their permanent level in handwriting during grades one and two, while poor writers learn at a slower rate (Karlsdottir, 1996). For handwriting to be easily legible, at least 50 percent of the letters must be mastered, and this takes place in grades one and two. The equality of children's handwriting should be expected to develop quickly during grade one and reach its permanent level during grade two. The speed of children's handwriting should be expected to develop approximately linearly with grades through primary school. There are numerous differences between functional and nonfunctional handwriters. These include:

1. Poor writers are characterized by longer movement trajectories.
2. Poor writers move faster and their movement trajectories are larger.
3. Good writers decrease average stroke length with increasing age, whereas poor writers produce increasingly larger trajectories when they grow older (Van Galen, 1993).

What factors are involved in children's handwriting and what causes deficiencies in children's handwriting? When a child is 7 to 9 years, you have an unstable period characterized by *ramp* movements (low, constant velocity of longer duration) and *step* movements (many composite submovements to the endpoint) until age 9, when the mature medium speed single-step movements predominate (Van Galen, 1993).

In general, every letter stroke is characterized by one major impulse that is associated with one velocity peak. In other words, one force impulse suffices to produce a letter stroke. This type of movement is referred to as *ballistic* (Karlsdottir, 1996). When a child is 5 years old, you see the first ballistic movements (short duration, high velocity, rapid acceleration and deceleration). Before the start of these movements, a movement plan has to be ready, and such a plan has to incorporate various types of information about the movement. One type of plan is about the letter form, in particular, the specification of the trajectory for the movement in space. The second type of information is related to the forces with which movements are made, which become manifest in the size, speed, and duration of the movements. Finally, muscle groups have to be specified and activated for execution. For example, a writer can either employ the finger/thumb in coordination with the wrist muscle system as is usually done, or in the case of writing with chalk on the board, use arm and shoulder muscles. A cause of deficiencies in children's handwriting may be the inadequate control of the various muscles involved in movement execution (Wann, 1991). Poor writing is not related to an information processing deficiency (cognition), but is a strategic phenomenon. Poor handwriting is the result of a deficient movement strategy (Van Galen, 1993). Handwriting is carried out with a variety of coordinated movements, and the child must be able to control spatial, temporal, and force requirements of the task (Maeland, 1992).

In the preceding sections, we have learned that poor handwriting is probably the result of poor motor planning, perceptual deficiencies, and poor coordination of the complicated fine motor movements that are required for adequate writing. This is one school of thought and is definitely the case for dyslexic and dysgraphic writers, as well as some normal functioning children with sloppy handwriting. Is it the case for all normal children who have sloppy handwriting? Recent and past research suggests that it is not and present another view. Research in 1981 found a weak correlation between the Bender-Gestalt Test (a form-copy test) and poor handwriting. Also there was no difference between good and poor writers on five fine motor tests. This indicates that normal school aged children on the average (not dyslexics or dysgraphics) have sufficient perception and motor abilities to develop functional handwriting (Karlsdottir, 1996). However, the production of handwriting at high speeds does require well developed motor abilities, and handwriting speed develops at the same steady rate for both good and poor handwriters. If it is not fine motor or perceptual skills that cause sloppy handwriting in some normal children, what is it? It has been shown that when formal instruction in handwriting stops, deterioration of the form aspects of the script occurs (Hamstra-Bletz, 1990). In fact, formal handwriting instruction often ends well before fourth grade. Children with functional handwriting at the end of first grade do not make significant improvements in their handwriting during the higher grades. Good handwriters reach their permanent level of handwriting during grades one and two, and this is when formal handwriting instruction stops. After grade one, handwriting instruction is often not repeated so poor handwriters are left to learn on their own (Karlsdottir, 1996). The use of special letter forms, certain cursive alphabets, practicing handwriting movements and tracing, do not greatly influence the development of handwriting. What does seem to help is the formal type of education that the children receive in first grade and the combined visual and verbal demonstrations prior to copying practice. It was found that the combination of visual and verbal demonstrations were superior to either just visual or verbal demonstrations, which were superior to copying practice without any visual or verbal demonstrations (Karlsdottir, 2002). Cognitive understanding of the letter forms and not perception, per se, may be of primary importance in the development of cursive handwriting (Karlsdottir, 1996). All children (including dysgraphic and dyslexic children) should continue to receive visual and verbal demonstrations prior to copying practice.

Another question that needs to be answered is why are boys more likely than girls to have poor handwriting? No one has come up with an adequate explanation for this; however, it is interesting to note that the ratio of boys to girls with poor handwriting in these grades (first and second) was three to one, while the ratio of boys to girls who have attentional problems is between three to one and nine to one (Karlsdottir, 1996). Could it be that boys more often than girls are not paying attention when formal handwriting instruction is given in grades one and two? So far, this question has not been answered.

There is a large difference between visual motor perception and sloppy handwriting. We train children in visual motor perceptual skills because many of the same skills that are required to adequately perform visual motor perceptual activities are also required for such school activities as reading. These include long- and short-term memory organization, understanding of the spatial relations of letters to each other, sequencing (also needed for phonics), directionality (overcoming reversals), ocular motor and visual scanning (needed for temporally processing letters in words and words in sentences), motor planning (the ability to cognitively form a plan of action), visual perception (to interpret and understand what we see based on past experiences), and coordination of fine motor skills.

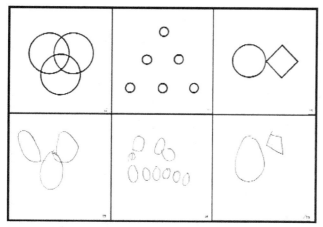

Figure 6-2. Examples of immature perceptual skills.

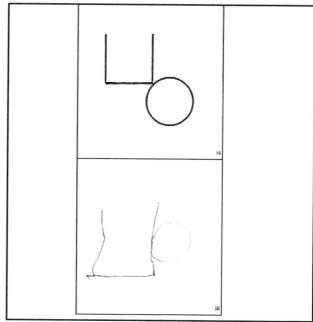

Figure 6-3A. Examples of poor spatial relations.

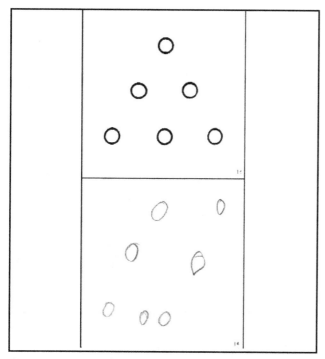

Figure 6-3B. Examples of poor spatial relations.

Training Tips

A. Be observant. You can learn a great deal about the child with whom you are working by observing him when he draws. Look for the following:

1. Holding his head close to the paper. This may be the result of the following:

   a. Inadequately processing somatosensory information and relying heavily on vision. The child may position his head close to the paper in order to visually monitor what his hand is doing.

   b. Poor vision. A child who is very nearsighted may have to hold his head near the paper in order to clearly see what he is drawing.

   c. Stress. Often children who feel very stressed while doing a visual motor perceptual activity will hold their heads close to the paper. They often will also lean on one arm as they do the drawing.

2. Poor pencil grip. This is frequently the result of a child trying to increase somatosensory feedback. The child may develop poor pencil grip characterized by stabilization of distal joints (Fisher, 1991).

3. Keeping his drawing in a vertical orientation. A child who turns his paper to keep the drawings in a vertical orientation shows immaturity. In spontaneous scribbling, a child normally produces vertical lines before he produces horizontal lines. A vertical diamond is expected by 7 to 8 years of age, whereas the horizontal diamond the norm is by 10. Only 61% of 6-year-olds produced the horizontal diamond adequately (Beery, 1982).

4. Immature perceptual skills. Figure 6-2 shows examples of immature perceptual skills.

5. These children show very poor spatial relations. At 5 years, you can start to expect the child to put the circle at the lower right corner of the open square (Figures 6-3 through 6-4).

This child shows directional confusion. Children who have these problems are often more likely to reverse letters when they print.

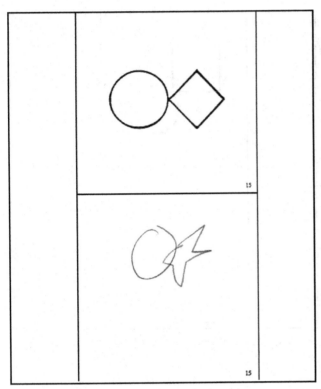

Figure 6-4A. Examples of poor spatial relations.

Figure 6-4B. Examples of poor spatial relations.

B. Know the developmental age of the child. Just because a child has a chronological age of 8 does not mean that his age in visual motor perception is also 8. For example, a child may be 8 years old but have a developmental age of 5. You would not expect this child to be able to draw a vertical diamond. You would have to start your training at a 5-year-old level. This means that you will need to do a developmental test to determine his developmental age. Each of the activities in this book is broken into levels of difficulty that will help you in determining a starting point.

C. Follow the normal developmental sequence when you do your training. The normal sequence of children's drawings is: vertical line (age 2 to 3), horizontal line (age 2 to 3), circle (age 3.0 to 3.5), vertical cross (age 4), square (age 4 to 5), triangle (age 5), directional arrows (age 6.5), vertical diamond (age 8), horizontal diamond (age 10 to 11) (Beery, 1982).

D. Follow the normal ontogenetic development of movement control. Have the child start with large drawings using more proximal muscles near the body. For example, using large circles keeping his wrist and thumb and finger immobile. Just have the child hold his arm out straight and use arm and shoulder muscles. Next, go to the more distal structures and have him just move his wrist. Finally, have him keep his wrist immobile and just use his finger and thumb.

E. Don't just rely on kinesthetic training (the movement of muscles, tendons and joints). Add cognition. Don't just show the child what you want him to do, verbally explain it as well.

References

Beery, K. E. (1982). *The developmental test of visual-motor integration*. Cleveland, OH: Modern Curriculum Press; 1982.

Broderick, P. (1987). The drawing of squares and diamonds: A perceptual-motor task analysis. *Journal of Experimental Child Psychology, 43,* 44-61.

Ellis, A. (1995). *Reading, writing and dyslexia: A cognitive analysis*. London: Hove.

Fisher, A. G. (1991). *Sensory integration theory and practice*. Philadelphia: F. A. Davis Co.

Hamstra-Bletz, L. (1990). Development of handwriting in primary school: A longitudinal study. *Perceptual and Motor Skills, 70,* 759-770.

Kapur, N. (1983). Dysgraphia for letters: A form of motor memory deficit? *Journal of Neurology, Neurosurgery, and Psychiatry, 46,* 573-575.

Karlsdottir, R. (1996). Development of cursive handwriting. *Perceptual and Motor Skills, 82,* 659-673.

Karlsdottir, R. (2002). Problems in developing functional handwriting. *Perceptual and Motor Skills, 94,* 623-662.

Kirk, U. (1981). The development and use of rules in the acquisitions of perceptual motor skills. *Child Development, 52,* 294-305.

Kopptiz, E. M. (1963). *The Bender Gestalt test for young children.* Orlando, FL: Grune and Stratton, Inc.

Levinson, H. N. (1980). *A solution to the riddle dyslexia.* New York: Springer-Verlag.

Maeland, A. F. (1992). Handwriting and perceptual-motor skills in clumsy dysgraphic, and "normal" children. *Perceptual and Motor Skills, 75,* 1207-1217.

Mati-Zissi, H. (1998). Drawing performance in children with special learning difficulties. *Perceptual and Motor Skills, 87,* 487-497.

Mati-Zissi, H. (2001). Drawing performances of special learning difficulties of kindergarten children. *Perceptual and Motor Skills, 92,* 1154-1165.

Piaget, J. (1948). *The child's conception of space.* London: Routledge and Kegan Paul, Ltd.

Richards, R. G. (1999). *The source for dyslexia and dysgraphia.* East Moline, IL: Linqui Systems.

Strauss, R. N. (1979). Assessment of individual motor skills activities manual. Austin, TX: Education Service Center; 188-192.

Thomas, G. V. (1990). *An introduction to the psychology of children's drawings.* New York: New York University Press.

Van Galen, G. P. (1993). Neuromotor noise and poor handwriting in children. *Acta Psychologica, 82,* 161-178.

Wann, J. (1991). *Development of graphic skills.* San Diego, CA: Academic Press.

Form VMP-1
Bean Counting

Purpose: Visual motor.

Materials: Pint size jar filled with dried lima beans, tin can, metronome.

Method: Have the child do the following activities.

Level 1:
1. Have the child pick out 50 beans with his right hand and place them in the tin can as you count to 50 for him.
2. Spread the beans on the table and with his left hand, have the child put them back in the jar. Repeat using the right hand.
3. Have him pick out 50 beans alternating between the right and the left hand as fast as he can and put them on the table.

Level 2: At the beat of a metronome, he is to alternate his hands and take the beans out of the can and put them on the table. He then puts them back. You may increase the metronome speed but make sure he only touches the beans each time he hears the metronome beat.

Form VMP-2
NUTS AND BOLTS

Purpose: Visual motor perception.

Materials: Nuts and bolts of various sizes.

Method: Have the child do the following activities.

Level 1: Have the child remove all the nuts from the bolts. Mix them up and have the child put the nuts back on the bolts as quickly as possible.

Level 2: Have the child do the same as Level 1, but with his eyes closed.

Form VMP-3
LINE DRAWING

Purpose: Visual motor perception.

Materials: Blackboard.

Method: Have the child experience parts of geometric shapes by drawing the following on the blackboard.
1. Lines going uphill
2. Lines going downhill
3. Lines that start at the left edge and go to the right edge
4. Lines near the top and near the bottom
5. Diagonal lines
6. Lines that crisscross
7. Lines that bump each other
8. Curved lines
9. Circles

Level 1:
1. The child should use his right hand first and then his left.
2. Show the child how letters can be formed from these various lines.

Form VMP-4
FLASHLIGHT ACTIVITIES

Purpose: Visual motor perception.

Materials: Two flashlights.

Method: Turn the lights in the room down. You don't want it completely dark.

Level 1:
1. Name an object in the room. See how quickly the child can push the "on" button, aim the flashlight, and shine on the object.
2. Have the child move the light in circles and other figure patterns on the wall. Do first with his right hand and then with his left.

Level 2: Both you and the child have a flashlight. Shine your light on the wall in different geometric shapes or number or letter patterns. The child must keep his light on yours. When you have finished, ask him what pattern, number, or letter you drew with your light.

Form VMP-5
ANGLES AND OBLIQUE LINES

Purpose: Angles and obliques are the most difficult parts of a shape for a child to master. He must be competent at angles and obliques before he can master geometric shapes and letters.

Materials: Marker board.

Method: Have the child stand in front of the board. You draw an angle or oblique on the right side of the board. He must reproduce it as closely as he can. The parts of the angles must be in correct dimensions to each other. Also, the angle should be as close to the correct angle as possible. It doesn't have to be perfect, but close. Start with the age that you feel is close to the child's developmental age. The age at which the average child can correctly reproduce the angle or oblique is above each example (the developmental age). Once you feel the child has mastered the particular angle or oblique, proceed to "Proximal and Distal Kinesthetic Reinforcement" (Form VMP-6) and have him learn the enclosed shape that corresponds to the angle he has been practicing. It is very important that before the child attempts the drawing that you have him do the kinesthetic movements of the angle or oblique first. Take his hand and in the air show him the proper movements for each angle. Spend some time on this. I suggest 10 minutes, as a couple of minutes is not enough. As a variation, have him do it with his eyes opened and closed. He could also try it standing or seated.

Levels 1 to 5:

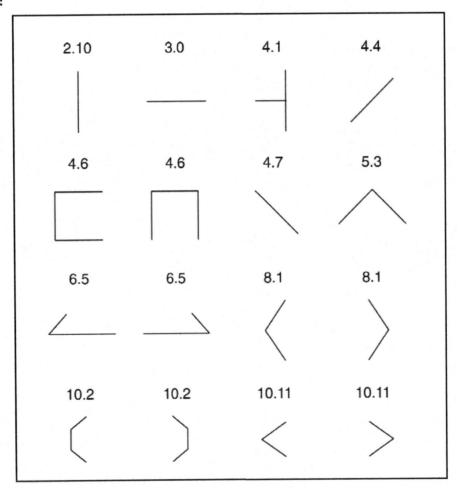

Form VMP-6
PROXIMAL AND DISTAL KINESTHETIC REINFORCEMENT

Purpose: To follow the developmental trend in copying shapes using kinesthetic reinforcement.

Materials: Marker board, paper, and pencils.

Methods: Method A
Use the following geometric shapes. The developmental age is above each shape. The developmental age is the age at which the average child can draw the shape.

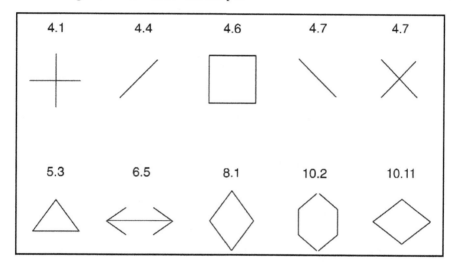

1. There are no levels in this activity. Start with the shape that is appropriate for the child's developmental age. Do all of the shapes up to and including the one for your child's age. When these are completed correctly, proceed to the more advanced shapes. It is important for this activity that the shapes are reproduced accurately. The lines must be the correct and appropriate lengths, the orientation of the shape must be correct and the angles must be as close to the correct degrees as possible. For example, a 90 degree angle should not be a 45 degree angle, etc.
2. Proximal Training—Have the child stand in front of the board. You draw the shape on the board. The child is to hold his arm out straight in front of him. He is not to bend his wrist.

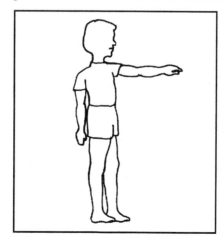

Form VMP-6 (continued)
PROXIMAL AND DISTAL KINESTHETIC REINFORCEMENT

Before he draws on the board, do 10 minutes of kinesthetic training. You move his arm in the correct movements to reproduce the shape. Do this with his eyes open and closed. Then, with his eyes open, the child draws the shape on the board. He draws it with his arm straight and does not move his wrist.

3. Distal (A) Do the same as proximal. However, now the child keeps his arm straight and only moves his wrist to reproduce the shapes on the board. Practice the kinesthetic training by moving his wrist in the proper directions to reproduce the shape.

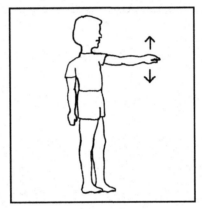

4. Distal (B) Now the child sits at a table and draws the shapes on paper by just moving his thumb and fingers. No kinesthetic training is needed for this exercise.

Method B
Do the same sequence of proximal and distal as in Method A, but now you make up shapes for him to copy. The following are some examples:

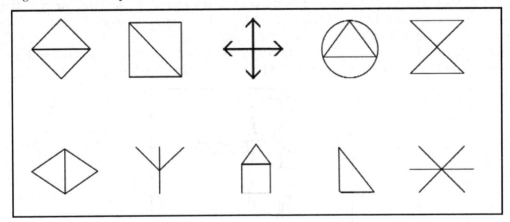

Form VMP-7
MOTOR PLANNING

Purpose: To develop motor planning skills.

Materials: Marker board, paper, and pencil.

Methods: The child is to copy the shape by either filling in the lines or using the dots as a guide to draw the line. The goal is to get the child to be able to draw it without any clues. Spend more time on oblique lines as these give young children the most difficulty. Have the child master all of the first group before he proceeds to the next group. Start by drawing the shapes on a marker board. When he has mastered the marker board, go to pencil and paper. Use your judgment as to how accurately the shape is drawn. Have him make it as accurate as possible.

Levels 1 to 3:
The child is to do all the drawings in Group 1 and then proceed to Groups 2 and 3.

Group 1: The child fills in the lines to finish the shape. You draw the examples on the board or paper.

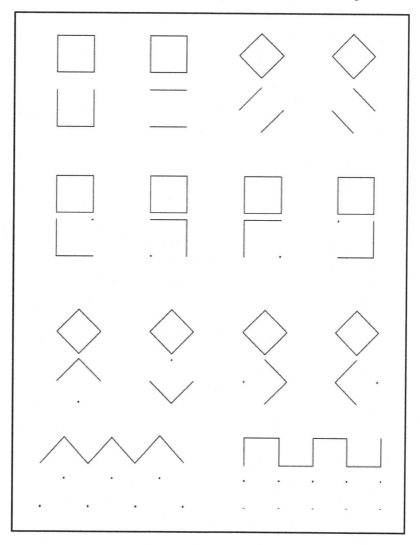

Form VMP-7 (continued)
MOTOR PLANNING

Group 2a: The child fills in the lines to finish the shape. You draw the examples on the board or paper.

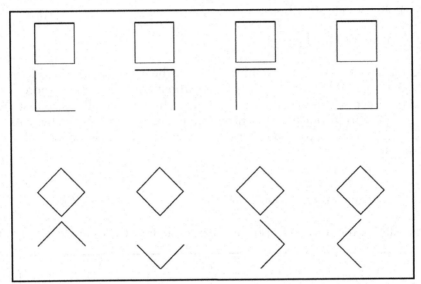

Group 2b: Same as Group 2a. The child fills in the lines to finish the shape.

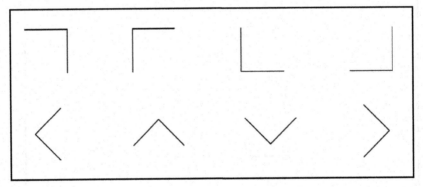

Group 3: The child draws the shape below the example.

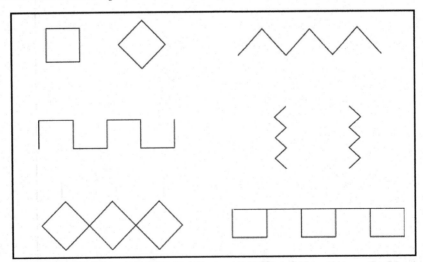

Form VMP-8
KINESTHESIA

Purpose: To develop kinesthesia that is critical for copying geometric shapes.

Materials: Marker board, sandpaper.

Method: Have the child do the following activities.

Levels 1 to 2: Have several geometric shapes drawn on the board. Have the child stand in front of the board with his eyes open. Show him the shapes. Then have him close his eyes. You take his arm and move it to duplicate the pattern of one of the shapes. He then opens his eyes and points to the correct shape. Do the same with sandpaper. The child sits at a table. You show him the shapes and then he closes his eyes. Take his hand and put his finger on the sandpaper. You move it to duplicate one of the shapes on the board. He then opens his eyes and points to the shape. For Level 1, start with circles or oblique lines. For Levels 2 and 3, add squares, diamonds, stars, triangles, etc.

Levels 3 to 5: After the child can do Levels 1 and 2, make the shapes more complicated. Also, make it harder by not showing the child the shapes first. He is to open his eyes and point to the correct shape.

Form VMP-9
FINISH THE DESIGNS

Purpose: Visual motor.

Materials: Marker board.

Method: The child is to finish on the marker board the designs in B to look like A. Do the following designs and then make up your own. For example:

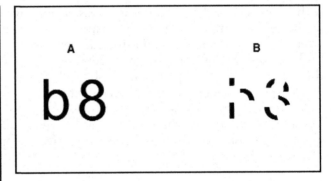

Level 1:
1. Do the designs above. Vary the missing parts. When the child has completed these, make up your own. Use as many letters as possible.
2. Draw the designs on a sheet of paper instead of the board.

Form VMP-9 (continued)
FINISH THE DESIGNS

Level 2:

1. Use the designs on the previous page in combinations. Vary the missing parts.
    When you have used as many combinations as possible, make up your own. Use as many letters as possible.
2. Draw the designs on a sheet of paper instead of the board, and have the child fill in the missing parts.

Form VMP-10
Geoboards

Purpose: Visual motor perception.

Materials: 2 geoboards, rubber bands, marker board. A geoboard is a square piece of wood 4 inch by 4 inch and 1 inch thick. Hammer nails in the wood so that they are evenly spaced and in rows. For example:

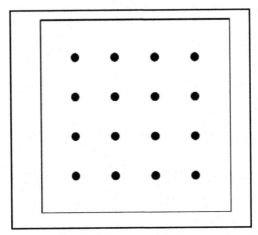

Method: To make patterns with the geoboards, stretch rubber bands over the nails. For example:

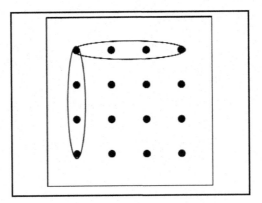

Level 1: Have the child copy on his geoboard the pattern you make with your geoboard. Do not use more than two rubber bands. For example:

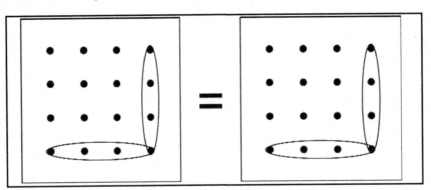

Form VMP-10
GEOBOARDS

Level 2: Have the child copy on his geoboard the pattern you make with your geoboard. Use up to four rubber bands. For example:

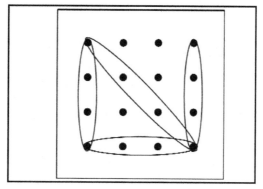

The child must use the same nails you use to make his pattern.

Level 3: Have the child copy on the blackboard the pattern you make with your geoboard. Use up to five rubber bands. For example:

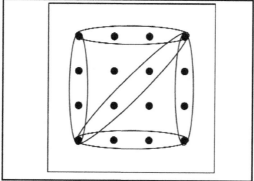

Put dots on the blackboard in the same pattern that you have on your geoboard. He must connect the same dots on the board as the nails your rubber bands cover.

Level 4: Make a pattern with your geoboard. Show the child your board for a few seconds and then hide it from him. He must remember the pattern and make it on his geoboard. Use up to four rubber bands.

Level 5: Make a pattern with your geoboard. The child must make the mirror image of your pattern with his geoboard. For example:

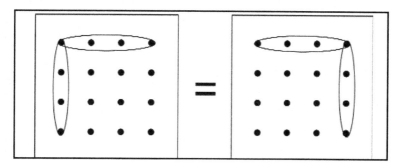

Form VMP-11
DOT PATTERN DESIGNS

Purpose: Visual motor perception.

Materials: Blackboard.

Method: Draw rows of dots on the blackboard to form a dot pattern. Draw a geometric shape by connecting some of the dots. The child is to duplicate your geometric shape by connecting the same dots with his own dot pattern. As you proceed from Level 2 to Level 5, you will gradually start to eliminate dots so that the child has less reinforcement to help him. When possible, have the child draw the shapes from top to bottom, and left to right. Have him describe the direction he is drawing each line. For example, top to bottom or left to right. Start with five rows of five dots. For example:

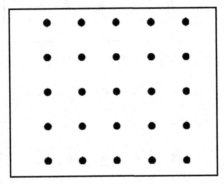

The child should be able to do the following geometric shapes in each level before going to the next level.

Level 2:
1. Make the basic shapes and letters as shown above. Use five rows of five dots. For example:

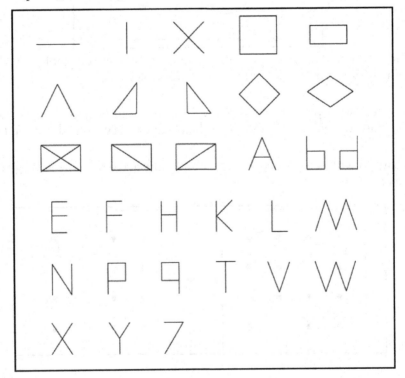

Form VMP-11 (continued)
DOT PATTERN DESIGNS

2. Make up your own shapes.
3. When the child can copy them correctly on the marker board, have him do it on a piece of paper. If you use paper, you will still use the same dot patterns for reinforcement.

Level 3A:
1. Make the basic shapes and letters as shown. Use the following dot pattern. For example:

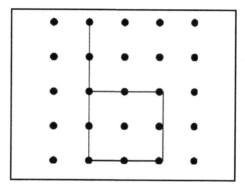

2. Make up your own shapes.
3. When the child can copy them correctly on the board, have him do it on a piece of paper.

Level 3B:
1. Make the basic shapes and letters as shown. Use the following dot pattern. For example:

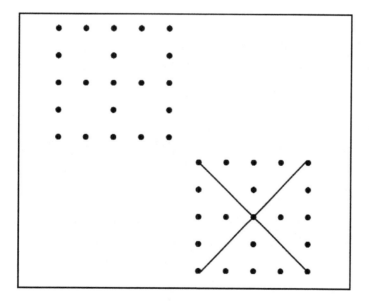

Form VMP-11 (continued)
DOT PATTERN DESIGNS

2. Make up your own shapes.
3. When the child can copy them correctly on the board, have him do it on a piece of paper.

Level 4:
   1. Make the basic shapes and letters as shown. Use the following dot pattern. For example:

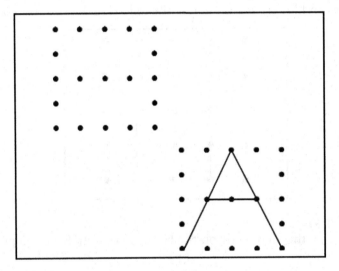

2. Make up your own shapes.
3. Have the child do the shapes on paper instead of the board.

Level 5:
   1. Make the basic shapes and letters as shown. Use the following dot pattern. For example:

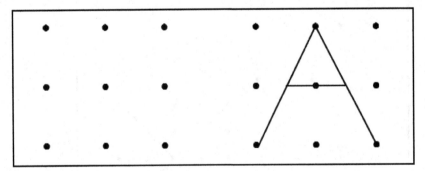

2. Make up your own shapes.
3. Have the child do the shapes on paper instead of the board.

Form VMP-12
CAN YOU IMAGINE A SHAPE?

Purpose: Visual motor perception.

Materials: Blackboard.

Method: Put some numbers on the board to form a pattern. Give the child a numbered sequence. He is to follow the sequence with only his eyes and tell you which geometric shape it would be if he drew a line in the sequence you gave him. If he has trouble doing it with just his eyes, let him use his finger and trace the sequence. If he still has trouble, let him trace it with a marker. Vary the number patterns. For example:

Example 1A:

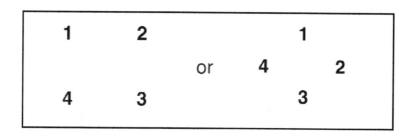

Sequence 1 2 3 4 1 would be which shape?

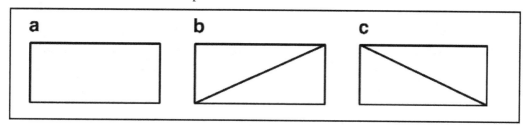

Answer is a, since the sequence is:

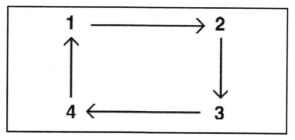

Example 1B:
Sequence 1 3 4 would be which of these shapes?

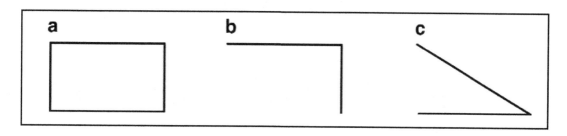

Form VMP-12 (continued)
CAN YOU IMAGINE A SHAPE?

Answer is c, since sequence is:

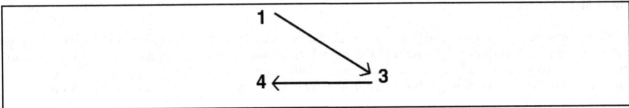

Level 2: Have the child trace the sequence with a marker and then point to the correct shape. Use a maximum of four numbers.

Level 3: Have the child trace the sequence in the air with his finger and tell you the correct shape. If he has difficulty, let him trace it with a marker on the marker board. Use a maximum of 5 numbers. Vary the number patterns. For example:

	1	2			1	2	3
5			3	or			
	4				5	4	

Level 4: Have the child trace the pattern with his eyes only and identify the correct shape. If he has difficulty, let him trace it in the air with his finger. Use a maximum of 5 numbers. For example:

1		2
	5	
4		3

Form VMP-12 (continued)
CAN YOU IMAGINE A SHAPE?

Level 5: Have the child trace the pattern with his eyes only and identify the correct shape. Use a maximum of 6 numbers. Vary the number pattern.

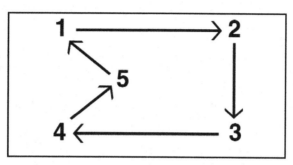

Form VMP-13
MATCHSTICKS

Purpose: Develop visual motor perceptual skills.

Materials: Matchsticks with the heads broken off. Always offer more matchsticks than are needed for each exercise.

Method: The child is to reproduce geometric shapes using matchsticks. You draw what you want him to reproduce. He is not to go on to the next level until he is competent at the level on which he is working.

Level 1: Have the child make a straight line. Have him make several straight lines of different lengths. Have him do oblique lines.

Level 2: Do Level 1 and now have him do the following:

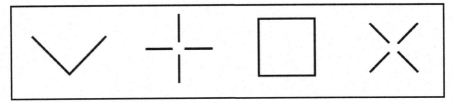

Level 3: Do Levels 1 and 2 and the following shapes:

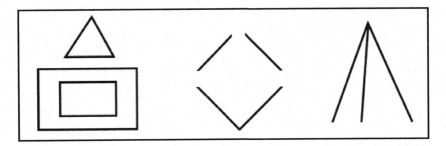

Form VMP-13 (continued)
MATCHSTICKS

Levels 4 and 5: Do Levels 1 to 3 and the following. Then make up your own shapes.

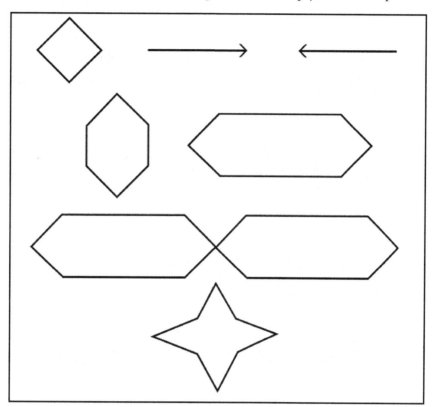

Form VMP-14
LINES AND SHAPES

Purpose: Develop spatial relationships.

Materials: Marker board.

Method: On a marker board, draw a geometric shape (see below) as accurately as you can.

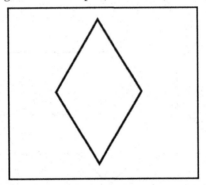

Have four groups of lines for the child to choose from. Ask him which set of lines will make the shape. For example, set "D" in the four groups below makes the shape above.

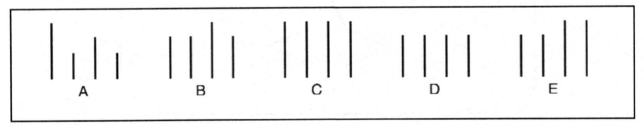

Vary the shapes. For example:

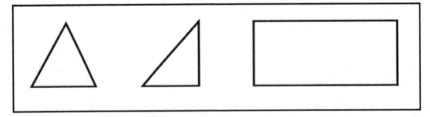

Levels 1 to 2: Have the child do the basic shapes as shown above. Create some new shapes.

Level 3: Have the child do the basic shapes, but after you show him the shape on the board, hide it from him and make him identify the correct line group from memory.

Level 4: Draw the shape on the board. Let the child look at it and then hide it from him. Have him identify the correct line group and then draw the shape as accurately as he can on paper.

Form VMP-15
ROUND PAPER DRAWINGS

Purpose: To eliminate any vertical or horizontal clues when drawing geometric shapes. There are some people who feel that children use the vertical or horizontal margins of the paper to assist them when they draw geometric shapes.

Materials: Take a piece of paper and cut it into a round shape.

Methods: Have the child do the following activities.

Levels 1 to 5: Have the child draw different geometric shapes that are appropriate for his developmental age. Draw the shape on a regular piece of paper and he draws it on the round paper. The drawings should be in proper alignment with the imagery horizontal line. For example, this would be appropriate:

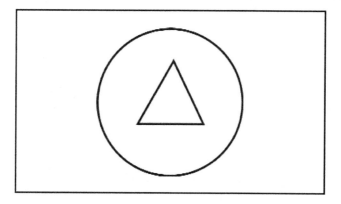

This would be inappropriate:

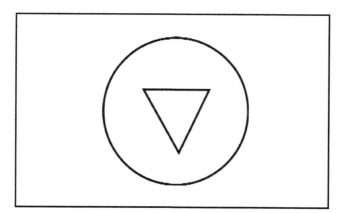

Form VMP-16
OCCLUDED VISION COPYING

Purpose: To develop kinesthetic skills.

Materials: Drawing paper, a square piece of cardboard.

Method: Hold a square piece of cardboard over the child's drawing hand so that he cannot see what he is drawing. Show the child what you want him to draw. He is to try to reproduce your drawing as accurately as possible.

Level 1: Do circles and straight lines. Vary the size of the circles.

Level 2: Same as Level 1, but add:

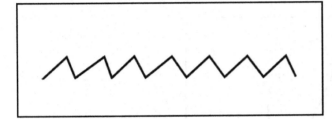 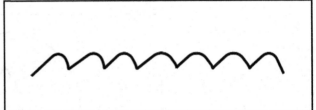

Level 3: Same as Levels 1 and 2, but add squares. Vary size of the squares.

Level 4: Same as Levels 1 to 3, but add vertical diamonds. Also have him alternate hands. First, do one shape with right hand, then next with left hand.

Level 5: Same as Levels 1 to 4, but add horizontal diamonds. Also make up shapes. Use shapes with a lot of oblique lines.

Form VMP-17
TRIANGLE AND SQUARE

Purpose: Develop visual motor perceptual skills and make him aware of directionality.

Materials: Marker board, metronome.

Method: Put an X on the board at nose height in front of the child. Draw a square and triangle on either side of the X. The square and triangle are about 1 foot in height. For example:

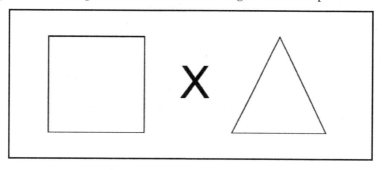

Levels 3 to 5: Have the child trace the lines of each figure simultaneously. The metronome is used but the child is not to name the direction of the hands, because one hand makes three different directional movements to complete the task and the other makes four. Have the child figure out the four different directions that the two figures can be traced.

Form VMP-18
BIMANUAL COORDINATION

Purpose: To train bimanual coordination.

Materials: Marker board, metronome.

Method: Have the child stand in front of the marker board with a marker in each hand.

Levels 1 and 2:
1. Have him draw straight vertical lines with both hands moving in the same direction at the same time. The lines should be the same lengths and both hands must move at the same speed. Continue this with horizontal lines. At each beat of the metronome, he is to draw the line. Set the metronome at a slow pace. At one beat, he draws it to the end of the lines. At the next beat, he goes back to the starting point.
2. Now add circles. Do circles in both clockwise and counterclockwise directions. Both hands must move at the same speed and both circles must be approximately the same size. You can use the metronome or clap your hands. At each beat he is to draw a complete circle.

Level 3: Do Levels 1 and 2, but now you call out clockwise or counterclockwise on the circles. He is to change direction at your command.

Level 4: Do Levels 1 to 3, but now the child draws one vertical line with one hand and a horizontal line with the other. Call out which hand you want vertical and which hand you want horizontal.

Level 5: Do Levels 1 to 4, but now the child does a circle with one hand and a line with the other. Call out, for example, vertical – right hand, counterclockwise – left hand.

Form VMP-19
CONTINUITY

Purpose: To make the child familiar with size differences and spatial relationships.

Materials: Marker board, pencil, and paper.

Methods: Have the child do the following activities.

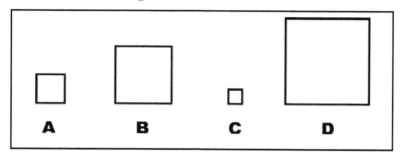

Level 1: Show him the four squares. Pick one and have him draw it the same size.

Level 2: Have him draw a square "bigger than" or "smaller than" one of the squares. For example, draw a square bigger than A but smaller than D.

Levels 3 to 5: Same as Level 1 and 2, but add this type of instruction:
1. Draw a square half the size of D.
2. If you cut B in half and put it on top of D, what would it look like?
3. Draw A inside D.
4. Draw A connected to B, etc.
5. Make up your own instructions.

Form VMP-20
POINTS AND CONTINUITY

Purpose: Shows the child that everything is divided into its ultimate elements.

Materials: Paper and pencil.

Method: Draw a figure on a sheet of paper and ask the child to draw one next to it.

Level 1: Draw a square on the paper and ask the child to draw the smallest square he can next to it. Continue with circles or crosses. Tell the child to make it so small that nobody could make one smaller. On another sheet of paper, have him draw the biggest square he can.

Levels 2 to 3: Do Level 1, but continue with line segments. Have the child draw a line under your line, but ask him to make it half the size of yours. Continue with your line on one sheet of paper and his on another. Continue by asking him to draw half of a half compared to yours. Ask him to continue to divide it in half. When he cannot draw it any shorter, ask him what he is left with at the end.

Levels 4 to 5: Do Level 1 to 3, but now try to get the child to realize that a line is a series of elements and that everything can be broken down into its basic elements. Also, have him close his eyes and visualize a line as long as a football field. Have him visualize that it is divided in half, then divided in half again. Ask him to continue to visualize that it is continuing to be divided in half until it reaches the smallest element it can.

Form VMP-21
HANDWRITING DEVELOPMENT

Purpose: Visual motor perception.

Materials: Marker board, pencil and paper, Proper Stroke Sequence Chart (page 41).

Method: The child is to stand in front of the chalkboard and do the designs that are listed below. Allow the child to do each design as large or small as he wants. Observe body posture, grasp of the marker, rhythmical movement of arm and head, and size of the drawings. Provide help where the child is having trouble. Once the child can do these movements on the marker board, have him practice them on unlined paper. For example:

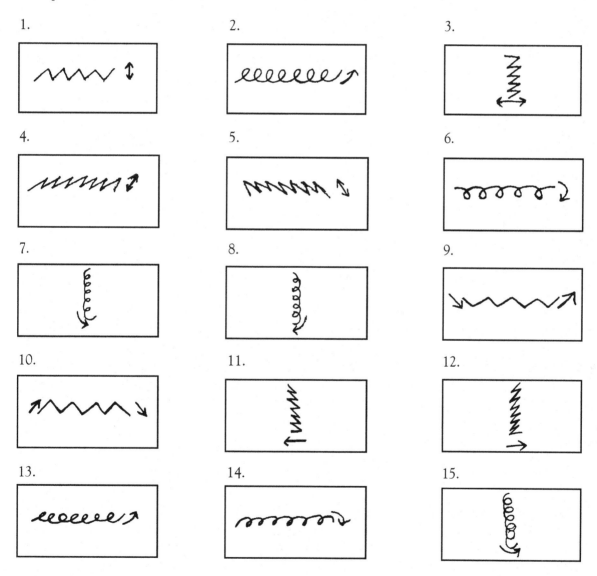

1.

2.

3.

4.

5.

6.

7.

8.

9.

10.

11.

12.

13.

14.

15.

Form VMP-21 (continued)
HANDWRITING DEVELOPMENT

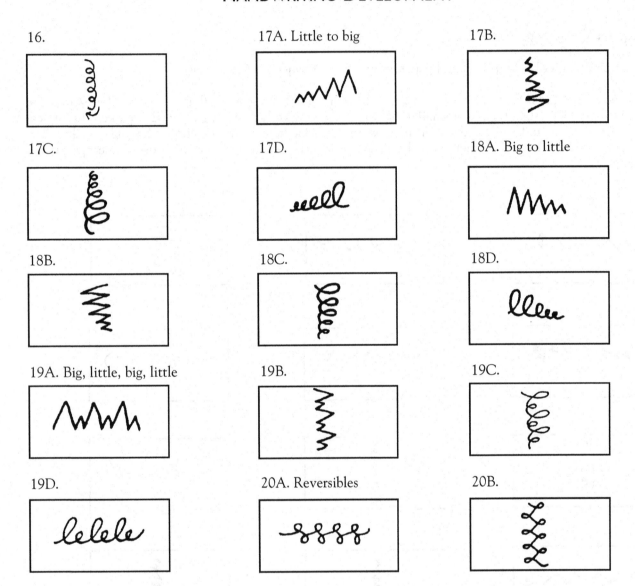

16.

17A. Little to big

17B.

17C.

17D.

18A. Big to little

18B.

18C.

18D.

19A. Big, little, big, little

19B.

19C.

19D.

20A. Reversibles

20B.

Level 2:
1. The child will do all the activities on the marker board.
2. Practice first with one hand and then the other.

Level 3:
1. The child will do all the activities on unlined paper.
2. Once the child can do all of the above activities, have him practice the proper stroke sequences for letters. Have him first draw the letters on the marker board and then on unlined paper. When he can draw them correctly on unlined paper, have him use lined paper.

Form VMP-21 (continued)
HANDWRITING DEVELOPMENT

Proper Stroke Sequence Chart:

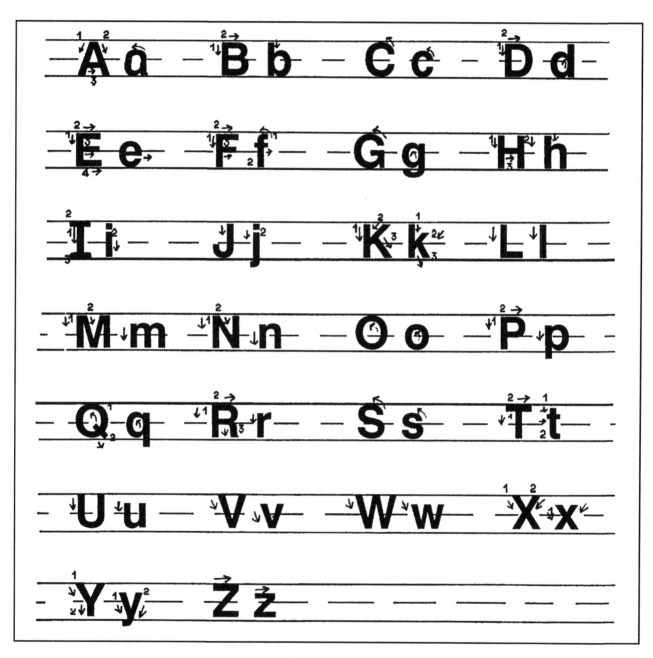

From Strauss, R. N. (1979). *Assessment of individual motor skills activities manual.* Austin, TX: Education Service Center; 188-192. Reprinted with permission.

Form VMP-22
LETTER SIZE SPELLING

Purpose: Develop size awareness of letters in words.

Materials: 5-inch x 8-inch index cards.

Method: Using lower case letters, make up three large index cards. One card will have all the "short" letters, one card will have all the "tall" letters, and one card will have all the "long" letters.

An example of letter spelling is as follows:
1. The word *read* would be: short, short, short, tall.
2. The word *pony* would be: long, short, short, long.
3. The word *yard* would be: long, short, short, tall.

Level 3:
1. Choose a category, such as colors. Ask the child which color is spelled with three letters and is spelled short, short, tall. The answer is red.
2. What color is spelled with four letters and is tall, tall, short, short? The answer is blue.
3. Continue with other colors.

Level 4: Same as Level 3, but use the other categories, such as animals, food, something to drink, etc.

Form VMP-23
FREQUENTLY DIFFICULT LETTERS

Purpose: To train the child to properly print difficult letters.

Materials: Marker board, paper, and pencil.

Method: These are the letters that children most often have difficulty drawing: **A, E, F, G, K, M, O, P, S**

Levels 1 to 5: Have the child master the above letters. Introduce the letters one at a time. Show the child the letter and verbally describe the letter. Do both upper and lower case. For example, a lower case f has a curve to the right on the top and a line crossing the middle. The letter M has two humps. After you show the child the letter and describe it, practice drawing it in the air and then draw it on paper. He will continue on this letter until it is mastered.

Form VMP-24
PENCIL GRIP RELAXATION

Purpose: Visual motor perception.

Materials: Pencil and paper.

Method: These activities are designed for the child who has a tight pencil grip or seems very tense during reading or writing.

Levels 1 to 3:
1. Have the child sit in a chair and at your command make a fist as tightly as he can. Have him hold it for the count of 10. Then have him relax his fist for the count of 10. Have him do this five times. Make him aware that he needs to relax while he is drawing or writing.
2. After he does #1, see how lightly the child can draw a line on a piece of paper. The object is to have him draw a line that is just barely visible.

Form VMP-25
Mirror Image Activities

Purpose: Visual motor perception.

Materials: 7-inch x 10-inch mirror, pencils, and paper.

Method: Two pencils are held together to draw a double line that looks like a racetrack (see Figure 1 below). Start with one or two curves with the lines not too close together. Later, you can add curves and narrow the track. The child sits looking into the mirror placed in front of him at a right angle to the paper and parallel to his body (see Figure 2 below). The paper with the track drawn on it is on the table. Try not to have the writing hand touch the paper, only the tip of the pencil. He is to move the pencil on the track from the beginning to the end without touching the sides.

Figure 1

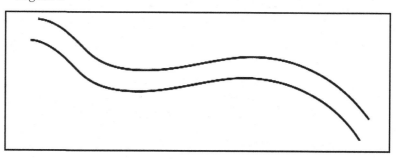

Figure 2

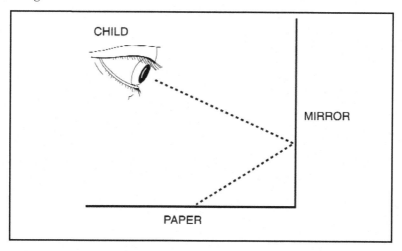

Levels 2 to 3:
1. The child is to look into the mirror and draw a line that stays within the track lines. If he goes out of the lines, he is to find his way back without lifting the pencil from the paper.
2. Turn the paper 90 degrees and have him go top to bottom.

Levels 4 to 5: Same as Levels 2 and 3, but instead of the track, put a series of dots randomly on the paper. The child is to connect all the dots. He must not lift his pencil from the paper.

Form VMP-26
Eye-Hand and Fine Motor Control

Purpose: Visual motor perception.

Materials: Pencil, worksheet with Xs and Os typed on it.

Method: With a pencil held so that only the point is touching the paper (no part of the hand touches), a continuous line is drawn over all Xs and under all Os in each line. For example:

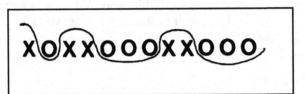

Levels 2 to 5:

1. Use the preferred hand. Be careful to draw the line in such a way that it does not touch any of the letters.
2. Use the nonpreferred hand.
3. Vary the activity by having the child underline every other group of Os, etc.
4. When he gets good at this, use a page from a magazine and have him draw over the first O and then under the second O and back over the third O, etc., until he gets to the end of the page. Time him. See how fast he can do this without missing any of the Os.
5. After the child can do the worksheet, have him do the exercises using other letters that are included.

Form VMP-26 (continued)
EYE-HAND AND FINE MOTOR CONTROL

O O O X X X O O X X O O X

X O O X X O O X X O X O X

X O X X O O X X O O X O X

X X O O X O O X X O O X O
Min._____Sec._____

O O X X X O O X O X X O X

X O X X O O O X X X O O X

X O O X X X O O X X O X O

O O X X X O X X X O O O X

X X X O O O X X O X X O O
                                        X
O X X O O O X X X O O O
Min._____Sec._____

Form VMP-26 (continued)
EYE-HAND AND FINE MOTOR CONTROL

VT - 1

X O O X X X O O X O O X X

O X X O O X X O O X X O O

X O X O X X O X O O X X X

X X O O X X O O X X X O O

O O X X O O X O X X X O O

O X X X O O X X O X O O X
Min._____Sec._____

X O O X X X O O X X O O X

O O X X O O X O X O O O X

X X X O O O O O X X X O O

X O X X O O X X X O O O X

X O O O O X O X X X X O O

O O X X O O X O X X X O O
Min._____Sec._____

Form VMP-26 (continued)
EYE-HAND AND FINE MOTOR CONTROL

VT - 2

X X O O X X X O O X O X O X X O O O O X X X X X O

X O X O X O O O O X X X X X X O O X X O O X X O O

X X O O X X X O O X X X O O O X X O O X X O O X X

X O O O X X O O X X O X O X O X O O X X O X O X O X O

X O X O X O X O X O X O X O X X O X X X O X X X O

X X O X X X X X O X X X X O X O O O O X

Min._____Sec._____

X O O O X O O O X X O O O X O X O O O O X O X X X

X O O X X X X O O X   X O X O X O X O X O X X X O X X

X O X X O X X X X X O X X X X O X O O O O X O X O

O X O O O X O O O X X O O O X O X O O O O X O X X

X X O O X X X X O O X O X X X X O O X O X X X O O

O O X O X O O X X O O O X X X O O O O X X O O O X

Min._____Sec._____

O O X O O O O X X X O O O X X X X O O O X O X O X O

O X X X O O O X X O O X X O O O X X X O O O X X O

X O X X X O O O X X O O X O O O X X X O O O X X X

X O O O X O X O   X O O O O X X X X X O O X X O O

X X O O X X O O X X X O O X X X O O O X X O O X X

O O O X X X O O X X O O X X O O O X X O X O

Min._____Sec._____

Form VMP-26 (continued)
Eye-Hand and Fine Motor Control

VT - 2

X O X O X O X O X O X O X O X O X X O X X X X O X X
O X X X X O X X X X O X O O O O X O X O X O O O
X O O O X X O O O X O X O O O O X O X X X X O O X
X X X O O X O X X X X O O X O X X X O O X X O O X
X O O O X X O O O X X O O O X X O O X O X O O
O O X O X X X X O O O X X X X O O O X O X O X O O

Min._____Sec._____

X O O O X X O O X X O O O X X X O O O X X O X O X
X X O O O X X O O X O O O X X X O O O X X X X O O
O X O X O X O O O O X X X X X O O X X O O X X O
O X X O O X X X O O X X X O O O X X O O X X O O X
X X O O O X X O O X X O X O X O O O X X O O O X X
O X O X O O O O X O X X X X O O X X X X O O X X X

Min._____Sec._____

O O X X X X O X O X O X O X O X O X O X O X O X X X O
X X O O X O X X O X O O O X X X X O O O X X X O O
O X X O O O X X X O O O X X O O X O O O X X X O O
O X X X X O O O X O X O X O O O O X X X X X X O O
X X O O X X O O X X O O X X X O O X X X O O O X O
O O O X X O O X X O O X X X O O O X X O O X X O X

Min._____Sec._____

Form VMP-26 (continued)
EYE-HAND AND FINE MOTOR CONTROL

VT - 3

```
O X O O O O X O X X X O O X X X O O X O X X X O O O X O X X X O O X
X O O X X O O O X X O O O O X X O O O X X O O X O O O O X X O O O X X
X X O O O X O X O X O O X X O O O X X O O X X O O O X X O O O X X O
X O X X X O O O X X O O X O O O X X X O O O X X X O O O X O X O X O O
O O X X X X X O O X X O O X X O O X X O O X X O O X X X O O O X X O
O O X X O O X X X O O O X X O O X X O X O X O O O X X O O O X O X O O O
```
Min._____Sec._____Horizontal
Min._____Sec._____Vertical

```
O X O X X X X O O X X X X O O X X X X O O X X X X O X O X O X O X O X X
O X O X O X X X O X X O O X O X X O X O O O X X X O O O X X O O O X
X O O O X X O O O X X O O X O O O X X O O O X X X O O O X O X O X
O O O O X X X X X O O X X O O X X O O X X O O X X O O X X X O O O X
X O O X X O O X X X O O O X X O O X X O X O X O O X X O X O X O X O X O
X X O X O X O X O X O X O X X O X X X O X X O X X X X O X X X X O X O
```
Min._____Sec._____Horizontal
Min._____Sec._____Vertical

```
O O X O X O X O O O X O O O X X O O O X O X O O O O X O X X X X O O X X
X X O O X O O X X O X X O O O X X O O X O X O X O X O X O X X O O X X O X
O O O O X X X X X O O X X O O X X O O X X O O X X O O X X X O O O X
X O O X X O O X X X O O O X X O O X X O X O X O O X X O X O X O X O X O
X O X O X O X O X O X O X X O X X O O O X X O O O X O X O X O O O O X O X X
X X O O X X X X O O X O X X X X O O X O X X X O O X X O O X X O O O X
```
Min._____Sec._____Horizontal
Min._____Sec._____Vertical

```
X O O O O X X O O O X X O O X O O O X X X O O O X X X O O O X O X O X
O O X X X O O O X X O O X X O O O X X O O O X X O X O X X X O O O X X
O O X O O O X X X O O O X X X X O O O X O X O X O O O O X X X X X X O O
X X O O X X O O X X O O X X X X O O X X X O O O X X O O X X O O X X X O O
O X X O O X X O X O X O O X X O X O X O X O X O X O X O X O X O X O X O
X X O X X X O X X O X X X X X O X X X X O X O O O O X O X O X O X O O O X
```
Min._____Sec._____Horizontal
Min._____Sec._____Vertical

Form VMP-26 (continued)
EYE-HAND AND FINE MOTOR CONTROL

VT - 3

```
O X O X O X O X O X O X O X O X O X O X X O X X X O X X O X X X X
O X X X O X O O O X O X O X O O O X O O O X O O O X O X O O O O X
O X X X O O X X X O O X O X X X O O X O X X O X X O O X X O O X O O
O X X X O O O X X O O O X O O X O X O O O X X X O O O X X X O O O X O
X O X O O X X O O O X X O X X O O O X X X O O O X X O X O X X X O O
O X X O O X O O O X X X O O O X X X X O O O X O X O X O O O O X X X X
```
Min._____Sec._____Horizontal
Min._____Sec._____Vertical

```
X O O X X O O X X O O X X O O X X X O O X X X O O O X X O O X X O O X X
X O O O X X O O X X O X O X O O O X X O O O X O X O O O O X O X X X X O
O X X X X O O X   X X X O O X X X X O X O X O X O X O X O X O X O X X X O
X X O O X O X X O X O O O X X X X O O O X X X O O O X X O O O X X X O O
O X X O O X O O O X X X O O O X X X X O O O X O X O X O O O O X X X X X
X O O X X O O X X O O X X O O X X X O O X X X O O O X X O O X X O O X X
```
Min._____Sec._____Horizontal
Min._____Sec._____Vertical

```
X O O O X X O O X X O X O X O O X X O X O X O X O X O X O X O X O X O X
O X O X X O X X X O X X O X X X X O X X X X O X O O O O X O X O X O X O O
O X O O O X X O O O X O X O O O O X O X X X X O O X X X X O O X O O X O O
O X X O O O X X O O X O X O X O X O X X X O O X X O X O O O O X X X X X
X O O X X O O X X O O X X O O X X X O O X X X O O O X X O O X X O O X X
X O O O X X O O X X O X O X O O X X O X O X O X O X O X O X O X O X O X
```
Min._____Sec._____Horizontal
Min._____Sec._____Vertical

```
X X X O O O X X X X O O O X O X O X O X O O X X X O O O X X O O X X O O O X
X X O O O X X O X O X   X X O O O X X O O X O O O X X X O O O X X X O O
O X O X O X O O O O X X X X X O O X X O O X O O X X O O X X O O X X X O O X
X X O O O X X O O X X O O X X X O O O X X O O X X O X O X O O X X O X O
X O X O X O X O X O X O X O X O X X O X X X O X X O X X O X X X X X O X X
X X O X O O O O X O X O X O O O X O O O X X O O O X O X O O O O X O X X
```
Min._____Sec._____Horizontal
Min._____Sec._____Vertical

Form VMP-26 (continued)
EYE-HAND AND FINE MOTOR CONTROL

VT - 4

k k g g y c c k r r b d d g g y j k k
q b p b d d b b p p q q b b d d p p
d d b j j p p h k h q q y b d c c y y
g g k k h k k h j j r r g g y y k h j
y g d p q q q b b d d p p p d d b b p
p d d b b d b b p p q p q b b d d p

Min._____Sec._____

q q b b d d p p d d b b p b d d b b
p p g g k k h h p q q y y c c d d r r
b d b b b d d p p d d b b q q b b d
d p p d d p b d d b b p p q q b b d
d d d p p d d d b b p p q q b b d d
p p d d b b p b d p b p b d d b b p

Min._____Sec._____

c c d d b b k h g g y y k k g g h h p
p p q q b b d d p p d q q d d p p b
q q b b d d b b p p q q b b d d p p d
d b b d d b b p p q q b b d d p p d
d b b d b b a a b b d c a y g k d p q
a j k j b q d y y g g j j k k h h p p

Min._____Sec._____

Form VMP-26 (continued)
EYE-HAND AND FINE MOTOR CONTROL

VT - 4

q b b d d p p d d b b p b d d b b p
p g g k k h h p q q y y c c d d r r b
d b q q b b d d p p d d b b p p d d
b b d b b d d b b p p q q b b d d p
p d d b b d r g g y r r y y h h k k j
j c c y y q q b p p q q r h k p d q g

Min._____Sec._____

d b b p p q q b b d d p p d d b b p
b d k k g g y c c k r r b d d g g y j k
k q b p b d d b b p p q q b b d d p
p d d b j j p p h k h q q y b d c c y
y g g k k c a c b b d y g h k y d a d
b a y c q k p b p b a b y d g k y g q

Min._____Sec._____

b b d d p p d d b b q q b b d d p p
d d p b d d b b p p q q b b d d d d
p p d d c c d d b b k h g g y y k k g
g h h p p q q b b d d p p d q q d
d p p b q q b a a b b d c a y g k d p
q a j k j b d y y g g p d h k p c q y

Min._____Sec._____

Form VMP-26 (continued)
Eye-Hand and Fine Motor Control

VT - 5

```
p d q b d q b p d q b p d q b p d q b d q b p d q b
p d q b p d q b d q b p d q b d q b d q b p d q b p
d q b p d q b d q b p d q b p d q b p d q b d q b p
d q b p d q b p d q b d q b p d q b p d q b p d q b
d q b p d q b p d q b p d q b d q b p d q b p d q b
p d q b d q b p d q b d q b d q b p d q b p d q b p
```
Min._____Sec._____Horizontal
Min._____Sec._____Vertical

```
d q b d q b p d q b p d q b p d q b d q b p d q b d
q b d q b p d q b p d q b p d q b d q b p d q b p d
q b p d q b d q b p d q b d q b d q b p d q b p d q
b p d q b d q b p d q b p d q b p d q b d q b p d q
b p d q b p d q b d q b p d q b p d q b p d q b d q
b p d q b p d q b p d q b d q b p d q b p d q b p d
```
Min._____Sec._____Horizontal
Min._____Sec._____Vertical

```
q b d q b p d q b d q b d q b p d q b p d q b p d q
b d q p d q b p d q b d q b p d q b p d q b p d q b
d q b p d q b p d q b p d q b d q b p d q b p d q b
p d q b d q b p d q b d q b d q b p d q b p d q b p
d q b d q b p d q b p d q b p d q b d q b p d q b p
d q b p d q b d q b p d q b p d q b p d q b d q b p
```
Min._____Sec._____Horizontal
Min._____Sec._____Vertical

```
d q b p d q b p d q b d q b p d q b p d q b p d q b
d q b p d q b d q b d q b p d q b p d q b p d q b d
q b p d q b p d q b p d q b d q b p d q b d q b d q
b p d q b p d q b p d q b d q b p d q b p d q b p d
q b d q b p d q b d q b d q b p d q b p d q b p d q
b d q b p d q b p d q b p d q b d q b p d q b p d q
```
Min._____Sec._____Horizontal
Min._____Sec._____Vertical

Form VMP-26 (continued)
EYE-HAND AND FINE MOTOR CONTROL

VT - 5

```
b  d  q  p  d  q  b  p  d  q  b  d  q  b  p  d  q  b  p  d  q  b  p  d  q  b
d  q  b  p  d  q  b  p  d  q  b  p  d  q  b  d  q  q  b  p  d  q  b  d  q  b
p  d  q  b  p  d  q  b  p  d  q  b  d  q  b  p  d  q  b  p  d  q  b  p  d  q
b  d  q  b  p  d  q  b  d  q  b  d  q  b  p  d  q  b  p  d  q  b  p  d  q  b
d  q  b  p  d  q  b  p  d  q  b  p  d  q  b  d  q  b  p  d  q  b  p  d  q  b
p  d  q  b  d  q  b  p  d  q  b  p  d  q  b  p  d  q  b  d  q  b  p  d  q  b
```
Min._____Sec._____Horizontal
Min._____Sec._____Vertical

```
p  d  q  b  p  d  q  b  d  q  b  p  d  q  b  p  d  q  b  p  d  q  b  d  q  b
p  d  q  b  d  q  b  d  q  b  p  d  q  b  p  d  q  b  p  d  q  b  d  q  b  p
d  q  b  p  d  q  b  p  d  q  b  d  q  b  p  d  q  b  d  q  b  d  q  b  p  d
q  b  p  d  q  b  p  d  q  b  d  q  b  p  d  q  b  p  d  q  b  p  d  q  b  d
d  q  b  d  q  b  p  d  q  b  p  d  q  b  p  d  q  b  p  d  q  b  p  d  q  b  p
d  q  b  p  d  q  b  d  q  b  p  d  q  b  p  d  q  b  p  d  q  b  d  q  b  p
```
Min._____Sec._____Horizontal
Min._____Sec._____Vertical

```
d  q  b  p  d  q  b  p  d  q  b  d  q  b  p  d  q  b  p  d  q  b  p  d  q  b
d  q  b  p  d  q  b  p  d  q  b  p  d  q  b  d  q  b  p  d  q  b  d  q  b  d
q  b  p  d  q  b  p  d  q  b  p  d  q  b  d  q  p  d  q  b  p  d  q  b  d  q
b  p  d  q  b  p  d  q  b  p  d  q  b  d  q  b  p  d  q  b  p  d  q  b  p  d
q  b  d  q  b  p  d  q  b  p  d  q  b  p  d  q  b  d  q  b  p  d  q  b  d  q
b  d  q  b  p  d  q  b  p  d  q  b  p  d  q  b  d  q  b  p  d  q  b  p  d  q
```
Min._____Sec._____Horizontal
Min._____Sec._____Vertical

```
b  p  d  q  b  d  q  b  p  d  q  b  p  d  q  b  p  d  q  b  d  q  b  p  d  q
b  p  d  q  b  p  d  q  b  d  q  b  p  d  q  b  p  d  q  b  p  d  q  b  d  q
b  p  d  q  b  p  d  q  b  p  d  q  b  d  q  b  p  d  q  b  d  q  b  d  q  b
p  d  q  b  p  d  q  b  p  d  q  b  d  q  b  p  d  q  b  p  d  q  b  p  d  q
b  d  q  b  p  d  q  b  d  q  b  d  q  b  p  d  q  b  p  d  q  b  p  d  q  b
d  q  b  p  d  q  b  p  d  q  b  p  d  q  b  d  q  b  p  d  q  b  d  q  b  d
```
Min._____Sec._____Horizontal
Min._____Sec._____Vertical

Form VMP-27
SPACE MATCHING

Purpose: Develop concept of distance.

Materials: A length of string, a steel tape, or a dressmaker tape.

Method: Have the child perform the following tasks. When he has completed each task, measure the distances and compare it to his estimate.

Level 2:
1. Ask the child to estimate the number of steps it will take him to walk from where he is standing to some object across the room.
2. Ask him to estimate the number of steps between two objects.

Level 3:
1. Ask the child to estimate the distance in feet between two objects.
2. Ask the child to estimate widths, heights, and depths of objects in the room. For example, pictures or window frames.

Levels 4 to 5: Have the child estimate fractional distances between objects. For example, 1/2 or 1/4 the distance between two objects.

Form VMP-28
3-D Tic-Tac-Toe

Purpose: Spatial relationships.

Materials: Pencil and paper.

Method: The child plays tic-tac-toe using three grids at the same time. Draw three tic-tac-toe boxes, lined up one in front of the other, for example:

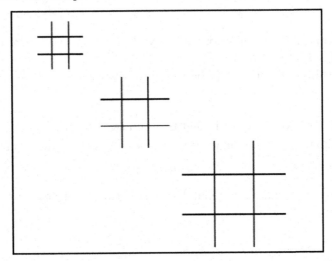

The child thinks of the three grids as being lined up like three light poles, one in front of the other.

Levels 3 to 5: The child is to play tic-tac-toe using all grids at the same time. For example, he marks an X on the first grid, you mark an O on the second and he marks an X on the third, etc.

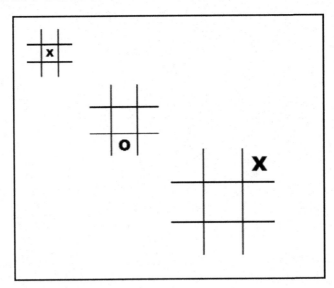

From Richards, R. (1988). *Classroom visual activities.* Novato, CA: Academic Therapy Publications. Reprinted with permission.

Form VMP-29
SPATIAL RELATIONSHIPS

Purpose: Spatial relationships.

Materials: Three colored blocks (the colors used in the activities below are yellow, red, and blue, but any three colors are acceptable).

Method: Sit opposite the child at a table. Place the three colored blocks in front of him.

Level 1:
1. Vary the locations of the blocks and ask the following questions:
   a. Which block is farthest from you?
   b. Which is in the middle?
   c. Which is closest to the blue block?
   d. What color are the blocks on the ends?
   e. Make up various questions concerning the locations of the blocks. Do not stack them on each other.

Level 2:
1. Have the child do the following activities with the blocks:
   a. Place the blocks on top of each other so that the yellow is on top and the blue on bottom.
   b. Place them so that the red is higher than the blue, which is higher than the yellow.
   c. Place so the yellow is in front of the red and blue behind the red.
   d. Place so the blue is on top of the yellow and red on top of the blue.
   e. Place so that the blue is lower than the yellow and higher than the red. For example:

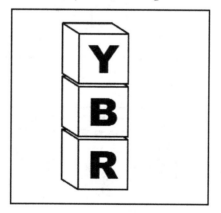

   f. Make up your own variation of the above activities.

Form VMP-29 (continued)
Spatial Relationships

Level 3:

1. Have the child do the following activities with the blocks:

    a. Place the blocks so the blue is lower than the red yet higher than the yellow. For example:

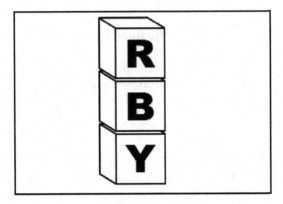

    b. Place the blocks so the blue is farthest from you with the yellow closest and red in the middle. For example:

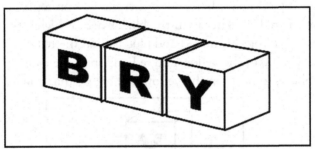

    c. Place the blocks so the red block is beside the yellow and the blue in front of the red. For example:

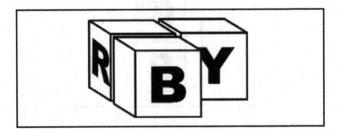

Form VMP-29 (continued)
SPATIAL RELATIONSHIPS

d. Place the blocks so the red block is to the rear of the yellow and the blue on top and between the red and yellow blocks. For example:

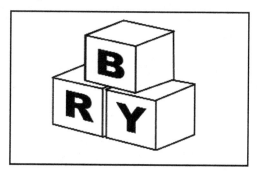

Levels 4 to 5: Make up variations of the above activities.

Form VMP-30
THE RELATIONSHIP OF "SURROUNDING"

Purpose: To teach the child the relationship of "surrounding".

Materials: Paper, pencil, stick, a ring that can fit over the stick, a string and colored beads, rubber bands.

Method: Will be explained at each level.

Level 1: Explain what "surrounding" is to the child. Give him the stick and ring. Ask him to make the ring surround the stick. Ask him to surround his wrist with a rubber band. Continue to vary this activity.

Level 2: Ask the child to draw one circle surrounded by another circle; ask him to draw two circles surrounded by one circle. Vary this exercise.

Level 3: This activity will use colored beads on a string. You will now work on the concept of "between". Have the beads on a string that is laying in a straight line. For example:

```
        O       B       Y       R       G       W       G
        O--------O--------O--------O--------O--------O--------O
```

1. Ask the child to describe the location of the yellow (Y) bead. The answer is between the B and R bead, or said another way it can also be between the R and B beads.
2. Ask about the locations of the G beads. Answers: one is between the R and W beads, one is next to the W bead. Both surround the W bead. You now can vary this activity using the concepts of "between" and "surround".

Levels 4 to 5: Do Levels 1 to 3, and now use a series of letters in a straight line, such as:

```
        A       B       C       D       E       F       G
```

We now need to have the child understand the concept of reversing a series.
1. Ask the child if C is between B and D. What else is it between? The answer is D and B.
2. If C is before D, E, F, and G, what else is it before? G, F, E, and D.
3. Vary this exercise using concepts of surround, between, and reversing a series.

Form VMP-31
LINEAR AND CIRCULAR ORDER

Purpose: To develop the concepts of linear and circular order.

Materials: Two strings of different colored beads.

Method: Have the child do the following activities.

Level 1: The child should be at least 5 years old for this exercise. You lay your string of beads in a straight line in front of the child. Have him put the beads on his string in the same order in a straight line.

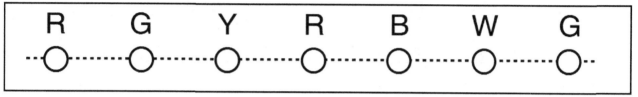

Level 2: Transposition of circular order into linear order. You make a circle of beads.

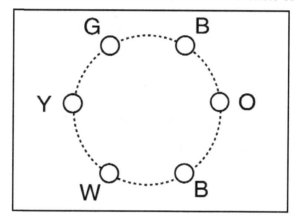

Tell the child to make a straight line of beads with the beads in the same order as your circle. Show him the starting point—in this case it could be the "B" bead. His should look like this:

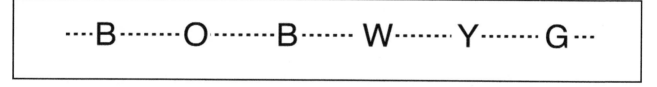

Form VMP-31 (continued)
LINEAR AND CIRCULAR ORDER

Level 3: Show the child a straight line of beads. Have him put his in reverse order. For example:

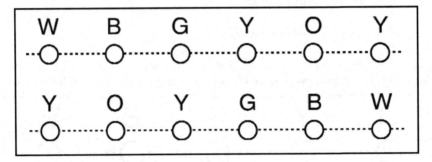

Levels 4 to 5: Show him a figure eight of beads. Have him copy in the same order. Start with the "B" bead.

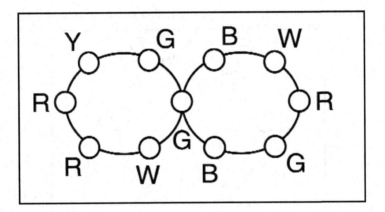

Form VMP-32
KNOTS

Purpose: To develop the relationship of "surrounding".

Materials: String or nylon cord.

Method: You show the child how to make the knot and he copies you. The child should reach the point where you call out the name of the knot and he does it without your help.

Level 1: Overhand knot. Form a loop by crossing the end over the standing part of the rope. Draw one end upward through the loop thus formed. This makes a solid knot when drawn tightly.

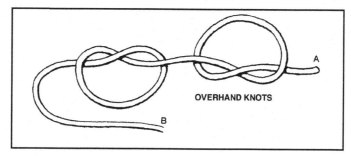

OVERHAND KNOTS

Level 2: Figure eight knot. Do Level 1 knot first and then this knot.

Figure 1   Figure 2

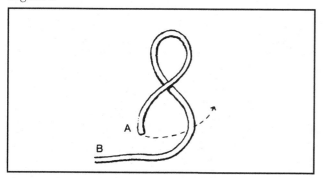 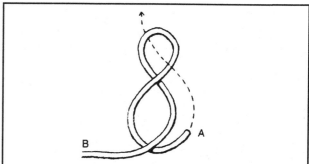

Bend the rope until it crosses the standing part, forming an overhand loop (Figure 1). Bend the end of the rope in the opposite direction to form an underhand loop below the first, giving the appearance of a figure 8 (Figure 2). Push the end up through the overhand loop and the knot will be complete.

Form VMP-32 (continued)
KNOTS

Level 3A: Square knot. Do Levels 1 and 2 and then this knot.

Figure 1

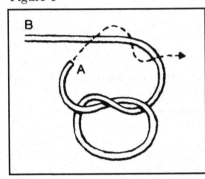

Figure 2

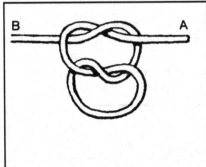

Figure 3

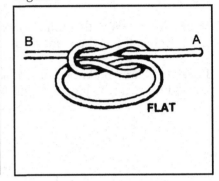

If you begin the first knot by forming an overhand loop, do the same with the second knot (Figure 1), or in other words, if you cross the end in front of the standing part to tie the first knot, do it the same way for the second (Figure 2). Pull the knot flat to finish it (Figure 3).

Level 3B: Bow knot. Begin with a simple overhand knot, then take a bight (a loop or slack part) in the standing part and tie the working end around it forming the second knot (Figure 1). The finished knot looks like Figure 2.

Figure 1

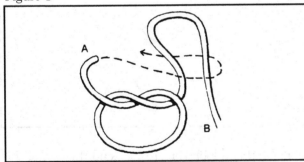

Figure 2

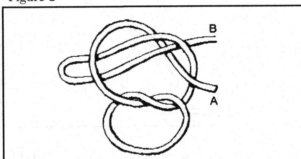

Form VMP-32 (continued)
KNOTS

Level 4: The bowline. Start with an overhand loop that serves as an "eye". Put end A (Figure 1) up through the loop, then under the standing part to form a turn (Figure 2). This brings the end over the standing part. Thrust the end down through the "eye" to form a bight (Figure 3). Grip both portions of the bight with one hand and pull on the standing part with the other. Thus the "eye" becomes a tight knot, below which you have a large loop.

Figure 1

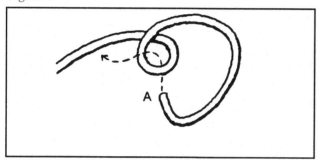

Figure 2

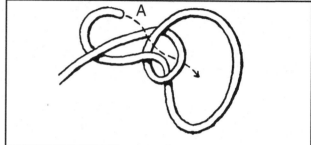

Figure 3

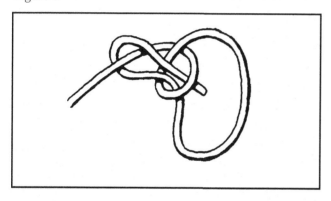

Form VMP-32 (continued)
KNOTS

Level 5: The shamrock.

Figure 1   Figure 2

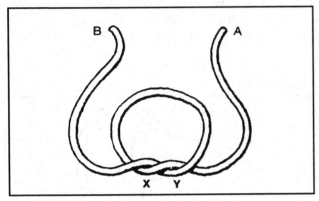 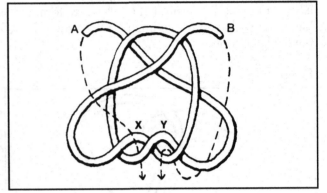

Tie a simple overhand knot with the loop above it and bring the ends up and above the loop one on each side (Figure 1). The end at the right ("A") is then carried toward the left and the loop is extended to lie across it. The end at the left ("B") is then laid across the loop toward the right (Figure 2). Pull the ends "A" and "B" straight down, tighten in the center of the shamrock, and at the same time, arranging the three big loops in uniform fashion to form the petals of the design (Figure 3).

Figure 3

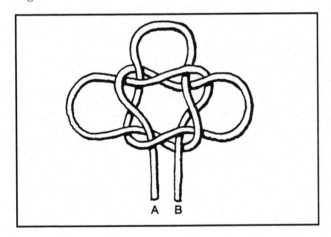

From Gibson, W. B. (1989). *Knots and how to tie them.* New York: Wings Books. Reprinted with permission.

Form VMP-33
VECTORS

Purpose: Directionality.

Materials: Marker board, protractor.

Method: A vector is a straight line at different angles. For example:

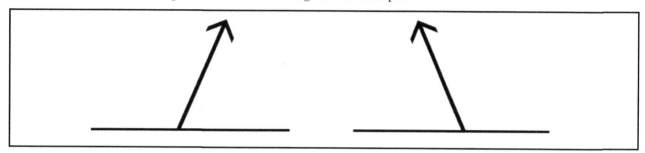

Draw several vectors on the board. Show the child how the angle can change between the vector and the straight horizontal line.

Level 2: Draw a vector on the marker board. Have the child draw one like yours next to it on the board. It must be close to the same angle as the one you have drawn. Draw several in different positions for the child to copy.

Level 3:
1. Make large letters on the board. Show the child how vectors can be part of a letter. For example:

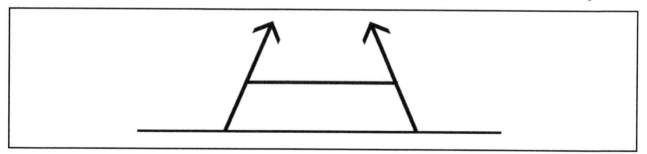

2. Draw a vector. Have the child make a letter out of it. For example:

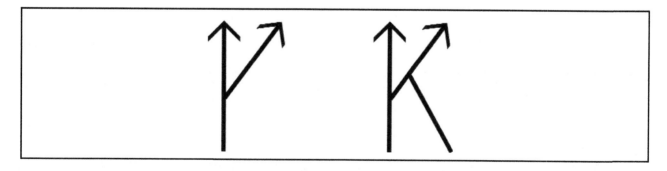

Form VMP-33 (continued)
VECTORS

Levels 4 to 5:
1. Draw a vector on a piece of paper with a protractor. Have the child make one just like it with his protractor.
2. Draw a vector on the paper with the protractor. The child must make a vector with the same angle but in the opposite direction.

Chapter Seven

VISUAL MEMORY

Memory results from the selective matching that occurs between ongoing neural activity and signals from the world, the body and the brain itself. (Edelman, 1998)

Parents of learning disabled (LD) children will often tell you their frustration with their child's ability to remember things. The child can remember what he did on vacation a year ago but can't remember the key words of a paragraph he just read. Why is it that a child appears to have a good memory but can't remember words from a paragraph he just read?

Philosophers have speculated about memory for at least 2000 years but its scientific investigation only began 100 years ago (Baddeley, 1990). The memory consolidation hypothesis proposed 100 years ago by Muller and Pilzecker continues to guide memory research today. The hypothesis states that new memories consolidate slowly over time. Newly learned information is disrupted by the learning of other information shortly after the original learning and suggests that the processes underlying new memories initially persist in a fragile state and consolidate over time (McGaugh, 2000).

The study of human memory is much more complex than just thinking of long- and short-term memories. Short-term memory consists of information that is maintained at a surface level of coding that is within the grasp of immediate consciousness or the focus of attention (Richardson, 1996). Short-term memory capacity is limited to 5 to 9 items (Weiss, 2000). When long-term memory occurs, a cell is electrically stimulated over and over so that it excites a nearby cell and if a weaker stimulus is then applied to the neighboring cell, a short time later, the cell's ability to get excited is enforced. Working memory is a central part of short-term memory and is involved in processing written or spoken language. Working memory does not hold and store information but is a system of temporarily holding and manipulating information as part of a wide range of essential cognitive tasks, such as learning, reasoning, and comprehending. It stores and processes information and then passes it on to long-term memory. Working memory can add to the long-term memory and the long-term memory can add to the working memory. The prefrontal cortex is the brain structure most closely linked to working memory (Dur Stewitz, 2000).

There is one kind of memory for pictorial information and another for linguistic. The recognition of pictures is essentially perfect. Such recognition is based on some type of representation in memory that is maintained without labels, words, names, or the need for rehearsal. Pictures are not stored as words. The image is received and stored permanently in pictorial form. Where words or other symbols are concerned, the first step of memory is to take the stimulus out of visual, pictorial form, code the items, and extract their meaning (Haber, 1970).

The hippocampus and its neighbors in the limbic system are way stations in the formation of permanent memories. The actual information is stored in the cortex, but for several weeks after it is first learned, it is passed around via the hippocampus. If it is recalled and used, more direct pathways develop in the cortex and the hippocampus is gradually excluded. If not recalled, it may be forgotten. If something happens to break the hippocampus connection, the information is forgotten. Without the hippocampus, learning is impossible (*Economist*, 1992).

History has shown us that there exist large differences in the memory capabilities of some people compared to others. Julius Caesar's memory was so superior that he could dictate four letters to his secretaries simultaneously. John Milton, who was blind, composed "Paradise Lost" in his mind, 40 majestic lines at a time, and then recited them to a scribe. Bill Gates, founder and chairman of Microsoft, amazes his colleagues with his ability to remember hundreds of lines of source code for his original basic programming. Aruro Loscami, conductor of the NBC Symphony for 17 years, knew every note of more than 400 scores from Bach to Wagner. At 87, he momentarily forgot a passage from Lannhauser in mid-performance. After he left the stage that night, he never returned (Parachin, 1997). When you look at these amazing examples of memory, you have to ask yourself: What is normal? Research has shown that the average adult, when asked to remember a string of numbers or the last word of each sentence while reading a text, remembered five (Lee, 1999). Most researchers feel that the most the average person can remember is seven. They call it the "magical number seven". That is, seven chunks of information is the most that the average person can remember. Most of us also feel that the best way to test a child's memory is to give him a digit span test, either letters or numbers, and see how many he can remember. It has been found that reading span correlates highly with reading comprehension, while simple short-term memory span such as digit span does not. In fact, digit span, the earliest and most commonly used measure of memory span, does not consistently predict the mainstays of everyday cognition such as reading comprehension (Losehky, 1998; Richardson, 1996). Another interesting fact is that short-term memory can be disrupted by irrelevant movements. This is obvious to a teacher who has worked with an ADHD student. Working memory capacity can predict performance in the following real world cognitive tasks:

1. Reading and listening comprehension.

2. Learning to spell.

3. Following directions.

4. Vocabulary learning.

5. Note taking.

6. Language comprehension.

7. Good writing.

8. Complex learning.

Broadly speaking, the most the average person can hold is about seven pieces of information. But if some of that information is visual and some linguistic the total increases (*Economist*, 1992).

Children with learning disabilities have problems in tasks that include being able to tell if words rhyme or taking a word and deleting the first phoneme and being able to repeat it. Several studies have suggested that differences between readers with learning disabilities and skilled readers as measured by reading, writing, and cognition functions are attributable to limitations in working memory. Learning disabled children were inferior in both verbal and visual spatial working memory (Swanson, 2000).

Dementia is an acquired persistent impairment in memory as well as other cognitive difficulties such as decline in language or visuospatial skills. Dementia ranges from 1% in adults at age 65 to 16% in those 85 and older. Prevalence rates double approximately every 5 years after 65 (D'Esposito, 2000). The risk of dementia rises with age, affecting about 40% of those over 80 (Lafee, 2002).

Mental exercise helps to stave off mental decline with age. People in the top 63% in mental activity had a lower risk of dementia than the bottom third.

1. Unfamiliar situations and challenges stimulate the brain; for example, try tying your shoelaces or brushing your teeth with your left hand if you are right handed.
2. Do crossword or other kinds of puzzles to stimulate your brain.
3. Talk aloud when you put down your keys or glasses. Tell yourself exactly where you put them (*Fort Worth Star*, 2003).

The main difference between short-term and long-term memory is that short-term storage retains words in terms of their sounds, while the long-term system retains words in terms of their meanings. Semantic information does not appear to influence short-term storage (McGaugh, 2000). Short-term memory capacity is limited to 5 to 9 terms (Weiss, 2000). Short-term memory consists of the information that is maintained at a surface level of coding within the group of immediate consciousness or focus of attention. Thus, short-term memory is a subset of long-term memory (Garzia, 1994). Stabilization of reverberating neural activity underlying short-term memory precludes long-term memory. This indicates that protein synthesis is required for consolidation of long-term memory (McGaugh, 2000).

Long-term memory happens when a particular neurotransmitter called glutamate is released. The formation of new synapses in active areas and the withering of those which remain unstimulated. Recent research suggests that this happens during sleep. In particular it seems to happen during the type of sleep known as rapid eye movement (REM). During REM sleep, people dream and one of the many explanations suggested for dreams is that they are like the film on a cutting room floor. The bits left over are experiences that have been waiting in hippocampus limbo and are edited into permanent memories. It has been shown that disrupting REM sleep also disrupts the formation of long-term declarative memories (*Economist*, 1992).

In order to get a better understanding of memory and children with learning disabilities, you need to get a better understanding of working memory. Working memory is part of short-term memory and deals with language processing. It has a number of subsidiary slave systems. These slave systems are:

1. The central executive, which is responsible for controlling attention.
2. The visuo-spatial scratch pad, which is responsible for setting up and manipulating visual images.
3. The phonological loop, which is capable of holding speech based information.
4. The articulatory control, which is based on inner speech.

Memory traces within the phonological store are assumed to fade and become unretrievable after about 1.5 to 2 seconds. The memory trace, however, can be refreshed by a process of subvocal rehearsal (Baddeley, 1990).

If the child repeats the word to himself (subvocal rehearsal), then he will insure that the word will stay in short-term memory and possibly long-term memory. It is interesting to note that the memory span for the phonological store is about 2 seconds. This means that the child can retain in working memory the amount of words that can be pronounced in 2 seconds. As you can imagine, this would be a problem for a learning disabled child who has difficulty with pronouncing words correctly or who is very slow at pronouncing words. In this child's case, he would have very few, if any, words in his working memory and therefore, not many will get to long-term memory. Short-term storage relies on phonological coding while long-term memory is more influenced by meaning (Baddeley, 1990). The problem seems to be that if the child can't pronounce it and have an idea of its meaning, it won't make it to long-term memory. This is why phonics rules need to be stored in long-term memory. Remember that working memory is a workplace, not a gateway. Information about phonics rules can reach working memory from long-term memory and help in pronouncing words and therefore, help get the words into long-term memory. Disruption of the contents of the visual state by irrelevant visual inputs can interfere with the phonological loop. Poor tracking, therefore, can prevent the child from gaining access to the passive visual store and adversely affect word processing.

Working memory is the mechanism responsible for temporary storage and processing information (Losehky, 1998). Even in the smartest of people, working memory capacity is limited. Researchers asked people to remember a string of five numbers or the last word of each sentence while reading text (Recca, 1999). The best performers could hold a total of five words in memory. Magazine readers generally decide in less than one-tenth of a second whether they will look at a page or turn it. Statistics show that headlines receive five times the readership of body copy. Text is usually read by only 10% (Lee, 1999). The brain decides very quickly if it needs to go and read the body of the text or skip it. When dealing with working memory, an amazing number of functions occur in the threshold of the mind. Messages and words are processed, a quick initial interpretation is made, and anything deemed irrelevant is pared away. Sensory information can reach working memory from new sources and from the long-term memory.

The phonological loop comprises a passive phonological store and an articulatory rehearsal process. Information in the store is subject both to decay over time and to interference from new verbal material. Loss of information from the store can be prevented by means of subvocal rehearsal. Also, by continuing rehearsal, the contents of the store could in principle be retained indefinitely. Operation of the store is impaired when it is subject to irrelevant speech. The disruptive effect is greater when the irrelevant speech is phonologically similar to the material already in the passive store. The operation of the phonological loop is limited by the length of time taken to pronounce the words for recall. Words of five syllables such as "refrigerator", "university", etc., take longer to say and are more difficult to recall than words of one syllable such as "salt" or "chair". The capacity of the loop is limited by how much speech a person could rehearse in 2 seconds (Richardson, 1996). The phonological loop is, therefore, linked to the speech system. From this information, you can see how difficult it would be for LD children to get words stored in their long-term memory. There are not many words they can vocalize in 2 seconds or less.

Just as the phonological loop is linked to the speech system, so the visuospatial scratchpad is linked to the control and production of physical ocular motor movement. Poor ocular motor skills will interfere with the visual scratchpad just as poor phonics skills interfere with the phonological loop.

The visuospatial scratchpad is a system assumed to be responsible for setting up and manipulating visuospatial images. The visuospatial system is somewhat analogous to the articulatory loop. Like the loop, it can be fed directly through perception (visual perception) or indirectly with the generation of a visual image. Recent studies have shown that some visually presented information accesses stored knowledge in long-term memory without necessarily being processed first by working memory. Remember, working memory is thought to be involved in visual-imagery tasks and in temporary retention of visual and spatial information (Richardson, 1996). Just as phonological loop is linked to the speech system the visual spatial scratchpad has been linked to the production of physical movement. If a child has very poor ability to control physical movements, such as poor ocular motor skills, then the visuospatial scratchpad will also be affected and it will hinder the movement of some words into long-term memory, just as poor phonics hinders some words getting into long-term memory. Children with learning disabilities are less able to generate pronunciations for unfamiliar words and are poorer at recalling visuospatial information compared with the good readers.

The third part of working memory is the central executive. The central executive takes information from both the visuospatial working memory and the phonological loop. The central executive could draw upon information stored in the phonological loop and in the visuospatial scratchpad to carry out further processing on the properties of the visual or phonological form of the word to allow spelling, segmentation, rotation of an image of the word, and so on (Richardson, 1996). The availability of a phonological representation of an item in long-term memory assists performance in a short-term memory task. It has been suggested that these long-term memory representations are used to reconstruct partially decayed short-term phonological traces.

Memory results from the selective matching that occurs between ongoing neural activity and signals from the world, the body, and the brain itself. The synaptic alterations that ensue affect the future responses of the brain to similar or different signals. These changes are reflected in the ability to repeat a mental or physical act in time and in a changing context (Edelman, 1998). This means that if you practice visuospatial memory activities, especially activities that use lines, angles or letter parts, then when real words get into working memory, they are easily handled and are easily formed into real words. An example of this is the Japanese language. The Japanese, as a group, score higher than American children on two visual recall tests (Sugishita, 2001). The tests are Visual Reproductions I and II from the Wechsler Memory Scale Revised (WMS-R) Test. These recall tests did not decline across age groups as much as the American groups. Both Japanese and English high school students know roughly 6000 to 8000 words. The Japanese use Chinese characters and the number of Chinese characters in daily use is approximately 2000, while there are 26 letters in the

English alphabet. The roughly 2000 Chinese characters take a tremendous effort to learn and write. Since the number of components in Chinese characters is 11 times that of the number in the alphabet, the effort required to remember these components becomes approximately 120 times that required to remember the alphabet. The Japanese are avid readers and the circulation of newspapers in Japan is the highest in the world—58% compared to 20% in the US. It appears that learning and use of Chinese characters has affected their abilities of visual recall (Sugishita, 2001).

Children's abilities to learn the novel, phonological structures of new words is supported by both their capacity to maintain verbal material for short periods of time and the use of existing lexical knowledge (Lafee, 2002). Abilities to repeat nonwords and to demonstrate good vocabulary knowledge are constrained by phonological loop capacity and by long-term knowledge of the language (Lafee, 2002). Several studies have suggested that the differences between readers with learning disabilities and skilled readers on measure of reading, writing, and cognitive functions are attributable to limitations in working memory. Poor readers were inferior in both verbal and visuospatial working memory (Swanson, 2000). We have to train the child in visuospatial tasks, and the school system needs to give the child the phonics skills necessary to succeed. If either one of these two areas is deficient, the child will have a great deal of difficulty getting the information to long-term memory and learning to read. You can train a child in phonics 8 hours a day for weeks at a time, but if his visuospatial skills are poor, he will not learn to read, and he will suffer frustration and failure in school.

Tips for a Successful Visual Memory Program

1. Teach the child to subvocalize when he learns a new word. He should subvocalize at least five times for each word.

2. Teach a child to remember long number strings by teaching chunking. For example, for the number string, 756134968, he should remember 756-134-968 or 75-61-34-968.

3. Find the child's limitation on the number of numbers he can remember. For example, if he only has a digit span of four numbers, don't expect him to remember more than four items.

4. Instead of remembering letter or number spans, try and get him to remember blends, short words, or pseudo words as they relate more to actual reading and comprehension.

5. Do the visuospatial tasks in the exercises given after this chapter. Don't do only language related memory training.

6. It is very important that you understand *expanded rehearsal*. This goes against the assumption many teachers and parents have that "massed practice" is best. Researchers have now found that it is much better to spread the therapy sessions out instead of giving a lot all at once. The strategy is as follows: a given item should be initially tested after a very brief delay. If the child correctly recalls it, then the delay should be systematically increased (a longer delay each time), whereas, if he is wrong, the delay should be shortened until he recalls it, then start to spread it out. For example, show a child a new word. If he is correct and remembers it, show him the word again in a half hour, then 2 hours, then 8 hours, then one a day, etc. You will get much more from a child if you spread your sessions out instead of massing them all at once.

7. Remember to test a child's memory ability to see if he will have school difficulties. Don't use digits such as single letters or numbers, but rather pseudo words or pairs of numbers to test his true memory ability to succeed in school.

References

Baddeley, A. (1990). *Human memory theory and practice*. Needham Heights, MA: Allyn & Bacon.

D'Esposito, M. (2000). Brain aging and memory: New findings help differentiate forgetfulness and dementia. *Geriatrics*, *55*(6), 55.

Dur Stewitz, D. (2000). Neurocomputational models of working memory; Nature. *Neuroscience*, *3*, 1184-1191.

Economist. (1992). The human mind: Touching the intangible. *325*(7791), 115-120.

Edelman, G. M. (1998). Building a picture of the brain. *Daedalus*, *127*(2), 37-69.

The Fort Worth Star Telegram. (2003) The new fitness regimen: Jogging your memory. June 26.

Garzia, R. P. (1994). Vision and reading I. *Journal of Optometric Vision Development*, *25*, 4-26.

Haber, R. N. (1970). How we remember what we see. *Scientific American*, *222*(5), 104-112.

Lafee, S. (2002). Mental blocked. *The brain in the news, 9*(1).

Lee, R. (1999). Thinking about thinking: Harnessing brain's power. *Communication World*, 20-21.

Losehky, L. (1998). What is working memory? *American Journal of Psychology, II*(4), 632-638.

McGaugh, J. L. (2000). Memory: A century of consolidation. *Science*, 278, 54, 51, 248.

Parachin, V. M. (1997). A good memory means success: Seven ways to sharpen memory. *Supervision, V5810*, 9-11.

Recca, L. (1999). Thinking about thinking: Harnessing the brain's power. *Communication World, 16*(9), 20-21.

Richardson, J. T. F. (1996). Working memory and human cognition. Oxford, England: Oxford University Press.

Sugishita, M. (2001). Learning Chinese characters may improve visual recall. *Perceptual and Motor Skills, 93*, 579-594.

Swanson, H. L. (2000). Are working memory deficits in readers with learning disabilities hard to change? *Journal of Learning Disabilities, 33*(6), 551.

Weiss, R. P. (2000). Memory and learning. *Training and Development, 54*(10), 46-50.

Form VM-1
IDENTIFYING DIGIT SPAN

Purpose: To determine the child's limit for digit span working memory that can be used for these exercises. Keep this in mind when you are doing memory activities. You want to push the child but not frustrate him. For example, if your child can only remember three digits in a sequence, you don't want him to attempt five. As your child gets better, you can expand his span, but you don't want to frustrate him in the beginning.

Materials: The digit spans provided in this activity.

Method: You want to show the child one digit span at a time. Start with three digits. He is to repeat back to you the proper digit span. They must be in the same order as the example you are showing him. Hold the digit span in front of him for the number of seconds there are digits. For example, show him a span of 3 digits for 3 seconds, 4 digits for 4 seconds, etc. He gets two tries. If he misses on the first try, show him the second digit span with the same number of digits. His digit span is the highest number he can remember in proper sequence.

7 4 2	**2 4 3 8**
8 1 6	**6 9 3 8**

Form VM-1 (continued)
IDENTIFYING DIGIT SPAN

9 5 3 7 6

8 4 9 5 3

Form VM-1 (continued)
IDENTIFYING DIGIT SPAN

6 3 2 4 9 1

1 6 8 2 7 4

Form VM-1 (continued)
IDENTIFYING DIGIT SPAN

6 1 7 3 4 5 2

8 1 3 4 9 2 5

Form VM-2
CLOCK MEMORY GAME

Purpose: Spatial memory.

Materials: Marker board.

Method: Have the child stand in front of the marker board looking at the X at nose level. Place eight numbers in a 12 inch to 18 inch diameter around the X like the numbers on a clock. For example:

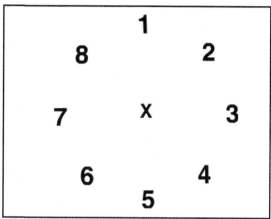

Level 2: Have him look at the numbers and then close his eyes. See how many he can remember and point to with his eyes closed as you call them out one number at a time.

Levels 3 to 5:
1. Same as Level 2, but call the numbers out of sequence, for example, 2, 6, 7. The child must remember and point to them in the proper sequence.
2. Same as #1, but use letters instead of numbers.

Form VM-3
AUDITORY SPAN

Purpose: Auditory memory.

Materials: Pencil and paper.

Method: Have the child seated at a table. For children 5 and under, don't use more than 4 numbers, and for older children, don't use more than 7 numbers.

Level 1: Call out numbers in a row and have the child repeat them back to you. For example: 5, 7, 6, 8.

Level 2:
1. Call out numbers in a row and have the child close his eyes for a few seconds, visualize them, then repeat them back to you.
2. Same as #1, but if he is old enough, have him write the numbers down after he says them.

Level 3: Call out numbers in a row and have the child repeat them and write them down. However, you are going to tell him to leave one of the numbers out. For example, call out "7, 8, 9, 6". Tell the child to say the numbers and write them down, but to leave out the 7. The child would say and write 4, 8, 9, 6.

Levels 4 to 5: For this, don't use more than 5 numbers and start with only 3. When he can do 3, go to 4, then 5 numbers. Call out numbers in a row and tell him to leave one number out and then write them backwards. For example, "4, 7, 6, 5" – leave out the 6. He would write 5, 7, 4.

Form VM-4
COLOR SEQUENCING

Purpose: Short-term memory.

Materials: Colored pens.

Method: Draw some colored circles in a row. For example: red, blue, yellow, green. Show the child the circles for a few seconds and then hide them from his view.

Level 1: Draw no more than three circles. Show them to the child for a few seconds. Have him tell you the colors in the proper sequence.

Level 2:
1. Draw no more than four circles. Show them to the child for a few seconds. Have him tell you the colors in sequence.
2. Have him tell you the colors in reverse sequence.

Levels 3 to 5:
1. Draw up to seven circles in a row. Have the child tell you the colors in proper sequence or in reverse sequence.
2. Have him tell you the proper sequence but he is to leave one of the colors out. For example, black, blue, red, yellow, green. Have him repeat the proper sequence but leave out the red. For example, black, blue, yellow, green.

Level 4:
1. Draw up to seven circles. Have him write the names of the colors in sequence on paper instead of calling them out.
2. Have him substitute one color for another. For example, every time he sees blue, he will substitute red for it.

Form VM-5
SEQUENCE MEMORY SKILLS

Purpose: Spatial memory.

Materials: Various objects in the room, metronome.

Method: Assign letters or numbers to different objects in the room. For example, the chair is number 1, the table is number 2, the lamp is number 3, etc.

Level 1: After you call out a sequence, have the child run and touch the objects in sequence. Do not do more than three at a time.

Level 2:
1. After you call out a sequence, have the child run to and touch the objects in sequence. Work up to 4 or more objects.
2. Vary this by having him run out of sequence. For example, 4, 2, 1, 3.

Level 3:
1. Label parts of his body with numbers. For example, #1 is his right arm, #2 is his left foot, etc. Have him move the parts in sequence. For example, #1 right arm, #2 left foot, #3 right foot, #4 left hand. You call out a number sequence. He then moves and calls out those body parts in that sequence.
2. Do to beat of a metronome.

Levels 4 to 5: Label parts of the child's body with numbers. Label parts of your body with letters. For example, you label his right arm #1, left leg #2, head #3, your right leg A, left arm B, and your head C. You call out a sequence and he then points to and calls out the proper sequence of body parts. For example, 2, 3, B would be his left leg, his head, and your left arm.

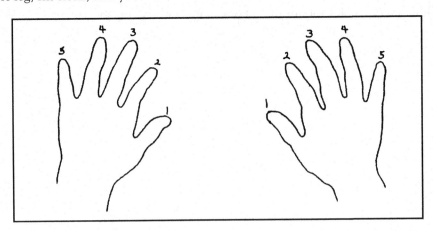

Form VM-6
RHYTHM

Purpose: Short-term auditory memory.

Materials: Metronome.

Method: The child is to reproduce the rhythm pattern. Sit opposite the child at a table.

Level 1: Beat out a constant rhythm pattern with one of your hands. Have the child look at you and do the same. Don't do more than a two beat rhythm. For example, da-dit, da-dit, da-dit.

Level 2:
1. Use a two beat rhythm and beat out a constant rhythm pattern with one of your hands. Have him look at you and do the same.
2. Same as #1, but have the child close his eyes and try to match your rhythm pattern.
3. Same as #1 and #2, but use a three beat rhythm, for example, da-dit-dit, da-dit-dit.
4. Beat out a constant rhythm pattern alternating between hands. The child watches you and repeats the rhythm with his hands. For example, R-L-R-L.
    a. Do double alterations, for example, R-R-L-L-R-R.
    b. Do three alterations, for example, RRR-LLL.
    c. Do irregular rhythm, for example, RR-L RR-L. Vary these patterns.

Level 3: Beat out a constant rhythm with your hands on the table. The child has his eyes closed. He is to figure out which hands are being used and uses the same hands as he copies the rhythm. Start with double alterations. For example, R-R-L-L-R-R, then three alterations R-R-R-L-L-L, and finally irregular rhythm R-R-R-L-L-R-R.

Level 4:
1. This is done with a metronome. The child is to touch his thumb to one of his fingers at the beat of the metronome. Assign numbers to the fingers. Have him touch the sequence you want to the beat of the metronome. For example, 2, 3, 4 or 2, 4, 5.
2. Use both hands. For example, 3, 2, 4 on the right and 3, 2, 4 on the left.

Level 5:
1. This is done with a metronome, with his eyes closed. The child is to touch his thumb to one of his fingers at the beat of the metronome. Assign numbers to his fingers. Have him touch the sequence you want. For example, 2, 3, 4, 5 or 2, 4, 5.
2. With his eyes closed, alternate hands. For example, 2, 4, 5 right, 2, 5 left.
3. Do #1 and 2 again, but with his eyes opened he is to touch the thumb of one hand to the fingers of the other.

Form VM-7
Hand Sequencing

Purpose: Motor sequencing.

Materials: None.

Method: Sit opposite the child at a table. He is to imitate the hand patterns you show him. P means palm down on table. S means side of your hand on table, F means fist on table. Show him a pattern. For example, PPS (palm down, palm down, side of your hand) and he does the same pattern with his hand. For levels 1 to 4, use only one hand.

Level 1: Do two patterns. For example, PP or SP and he then does the same pattern sequence.

Level 2: Do three patterns. For example, PSP or FSP or PPP and he does the same pattern sequence.

Level 3: Do four patterns. For example, PPFS or PSSF and he does the same pattern sequence.

Level 4: Do five patterns. For example, PPSSF or SFFPP and he does the same pattern sequence.

Level 5: Do four patterns, but alternate hands and he has to use the same hands and in the same sequence you use. For example, right hand PP and left hand FS, or right hand SF and left PS.

Form VM-8
DIGIT SPAN/SPATIAL TASK

Purpose: Stimulation of central executive.

Materials: Marker board or paper and pencil.

Method: For this activity, you must know your child's visual digit span. For example, if his visual short-term memory for digits is 5 digits, then don't use more than 5 digits for this activity. Draw a grid on the board. For example, use this grid for Level 1:

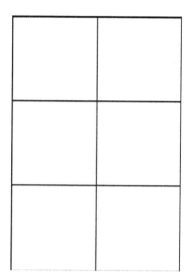

For higher levels, add to the grid. For example:

Form VM-8 (continued)
DIGIT SPAN/SPATIAL TASK

Level 1: Show the child your grid with a X in it. For example:

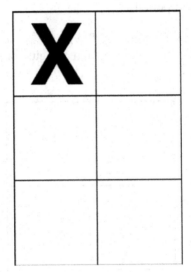

The child has a blank grid in front of him. You cover your grid and ask him to put a X in the same square in his grid that you had in yours. Go up to two Xs for this level.

Level 2: Same as Level 1, but increase the size of both grids and go up to three Xs.

Level 3: You will use the child's digit span for numbers. The child will put the same digits (numbers) in the same locations on his grid as you have on yours. Let him see your grid for 5 seconds. For example:

Form VM-8 (continued)
DIGIT SPAN/SPATIAL TASK

Levels 4 to 5:

1. Show him your grid with Xs in several locations. Then, show him a digit span of numbers. For example, 6, 4, 3, 1, 7. He remembers these digits and puts his numbers where your Xs are. Let him look at your grid and his digit span for as many seconds as there are digits. For example, 5 digits or Xs for 5 seconds, 6 for 6 seconds, etc.

2. You show him the grid. After you show him the digit span, he must remember the location of your Xs and his digit span.

X		X
	X	
X		X

=

6		4
	3	
1		7

Form VM-9
SENTENCE ENDINGS

Purpose: Stimulation of central executive.

Materials: Reading material.

Method: Have the child do the activities below.

Levels 2 to 3: Read the child several sentences. The child is to remember the last word in each sentence. For Level 2, read two sentences. For Level 3, read three or four sentences.

Levels 4 to 5: Have the child read several sentences aloud. Ask him to repeat the last word in each sentence. Start with four sentences and then increase the number of sentences. See how many he can answer correctly.

Form VM-10
DAILY MEMORIES

Purpose: Access to long-term memory.

Materials: None.

Method: Have the child do the activities below.

Levels 1 to 5: Use the same method for all five levels. The child's parents will need to cooperate for this activity. When the child comes into your office, ask him questions that pertain to his activities. Be very general for the lower levels and more specific for the higher levels. The following are examples of questions:

For the lower levels:
1. What did you have for breakfast?
2. What time did you get up?
3. What color is your car?

For the higher levels:
1. What was your mother wearing?
2. Who was the first person you saw at school today?
3. What color shirt did you have on yesterday?

Form VM-11
Motor Sequencing

Purpose: Sequential motor memory.

Materials: None.

Method: Have the child do the activities below.

Levels 1 to 5: Do the same type of movements for all levels, but for Level 1, only do two movements at the most. For Levels 2 to 5, do as many movements as was your child's digit span (which you found out in Form VM-1). For example, if he can remember 5 digits, do 5 motor activities.

Stand facing the child with your arms at your side and feet together. After each movement, return to this posture. You show the child a series of movements and he must repeat them in the proper sequence. He must also return his arms at his side and feet together after each movement. Some examples of motor sequences are:
1. Move your right arm out to your side.
2. Bend your head forward.
3. Lift up your left leg.
4. Bend forward at your hips.
5. Move both arms straight up.

Form VM-12
UPPER AND LOWER CASE

Purpose: Visuospatial scratch pad and central executive.

Materials: Chalkboard, paper, and pencil.

Method: Show the child a grid with upper and lower case letters. His grid does not have any letters.

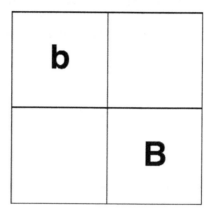

The child is to remember and draw in his grid where the upper and lower case letters were located. Show him the grid for the number of seconds there are letters. For example: two letters will be 2 seconds, six letters will be 6 seconds.

Level 2: Use a four square grid. Use up to three letters.

Levels 3 to 5: Increase the number of squares and the number of letters. For example:

b		d
	D	
	B	

Form VM-13
SEMANTIC ASSOCIATION

Purpose: Central executive.

Materials: Lists of words either on paper or on a chalkboard.

Method: Show the child a list of words. If he cannot read the words, say them aloud. He is to memorize this list. Tell him a word and ask him if it belongs in the list he has memorized. For example, pants, shirt, shoes. You say car, and he says it doesn't belong in the list. If you said sweater, it would have belonged in the list. You can also ask him if a certain word was in the list. For example, you say shoes and he says yes. Sweater would be no.

Levels 3 to 5: Some examples of lists are:
1. Car, bus, bicycle, truck
2. Basketball, baseball, soccer ball, tennis ball, beach ball
3. Grass, weeds, flowers, trees
4. Pencil, pen, chalk, crayons
5. Dog, cat, bear, lion, cow

Form VM-14
CHUNKING

Purpose: Short-term memory.

Materials: Paper and pencil.

Method: Demonstrate to the child how to chunk information so that it is easier to remember. It is just as easy to remember four chunks of numbers as it is to remember four numbers. For example, instead of remembering the number string 2 - 4 - 7 - 8 - 1 - 3 - 6 - 9, he should remember 24 - 78 - 13 - 69. Show the child several number strings. Show him how to chunk with two numbers each or three numbers each. For example, the above string could be easily remembered by grouping it into threes: 247 - 813 - 69.

Level 2 to 5: Have the child practice chunking. Start with four numbers and work up to as many as he can go. For example: 4789 would be 47-89, whereas 620145 would be 62-01-45.

Form VM-15
NUMBER SCANS AND MATH

Purpose: Central executive.

Materials: Paper and pencil.

Method: Show the child a list of numbers. He is to remember this list in the correct sequence. Before he repeats this list to you, have him perform a simple math problem. For example, show him 7 8 6 1 3. Before he repeats it back to you, ask him what is 12 minus 4? This is very difficult. You will have to start with a small amount of numbers. For example, start with just two numbers and work up from that.

Levels 2 to 5: Follow the method above. Start with two numbers to remember and very easy math questions.

Form VM-16
COLORS FOR DIRECTIONS

Purpose: Visuospatial scratch pad and central executive.

Materials: Chalkboard, pencil, and paper.

Method: The child is to move his X to get to the Y. However, colors are substituted for directions that the child has to remember. For example:

> blue = right
> white = left
> gray = up
> red = down

Show these to the child until he thinks he can remember them but not for more than a minute. Then show him the grid. In this situation, to get his X to the Y, he would call out:
Blue, blue, gray, gray, or gray, gray, blue, blue.

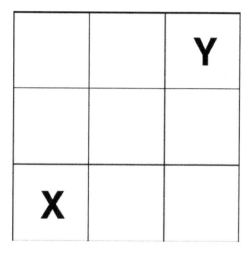

Levels 3 to 5: Vary the size of the grid and the location of the X; if the child calls out the wrong direction, move his X to that square and have him continue until he sees that he is heading in the wrong direction.

Form VM-17
Scan Memory

Purpose: Visualization and short-term memory.

Materials: Paper, pencil, chalkboard.

Method: Have the child close his eyes and visualize that he is going to move his hand. He is not to move his hand, just visualize that his hand is moving. Call out a sequence of several directions, and he is to visualize what shape his hand would have drawn if he actually moved it. For example, left, up, right, down is a square.

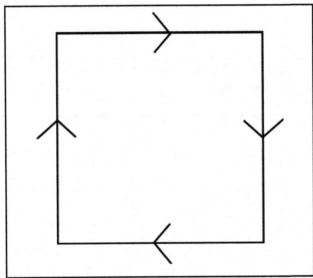

or left, up, right, up, right is:

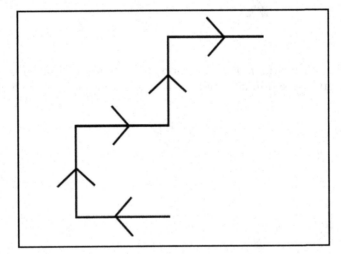

Levels 2 to 5:
After he thinks he has visualized it, have him draw it and compare it to what it actually should be.

Form VM-18
VISUAL SPATIAL MEMORY

Purpose: Visuospatial scratch pad and cerebellum activation.

Materials: Chalkboard, pencil, and paper.

Method: Have the child do the following activities.

Levels 2 to 3: Show the child the examples for 30 seconds and then take them away. Ask him what it would look like if the second figure was put on top of the first figure.

Level 3:
Ask the child what it would look like if the second figure was rotated clockwise or counterclockwise 90 degrees or 180 degrees and put on top of the first figure.

Levels 4 to 5: This time, don't show him the two figures. He has to imagine the two figures and what the result will look like if the second figure was rotated clockwise or counterclockwise 90 degrees or 180 degrees.

The following are examples you can use for this activity.

H + H = if 2nd H is rotated 90 degrees and put on top of the first H:

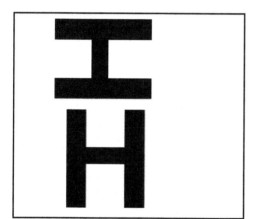

K + H = if H is rotated 45 degrees and put on top of K:

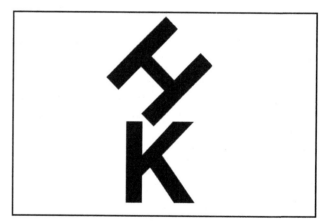

Other examples you could use:

B + B

A + B

L + D

J + H

You can also ask what it would look like if the first letter was rotated and put on top of the second letter.

Form VM-19
INITIAL BLENDS

Purpose: Initial blends are two or more consonants that are blended into a single speech sound. I consider this memory exercise to be one of the most important. With it, we are training blend sounds and working memory that will go into long-term memory and will be very helpful in learning to read.

Materials: List of blends, markerboard, or paper and pencil.

Methods: You will show the child several blends. Remember the child's limit on digits and work up to this. Show him the blends for 2 seconds per blend. For example if you have five blends, he will have 10 seconds to memorize them. He must repeat them out loud and in the correct sequence once you take them away from him. He must pronounce them correctly.

Level 1: See how many letters the child can remember.

Level 2: Work up to three blends.

Levels 3 to 5: The following is a list of initial blends you can use:

BL: black, block
CL: clean, club
FL: flea, fly
GL: glad, glue
PL: play, plug
SL: sled, slide
SC: scale, score
SK: sky, skip
SM: smell, smile
SN: snap, snow
SP: spark, spell
ST: star, step
SW: swap, swim
BR: brain, bread
CR: cream, crib
DR: dress, draw
FR: free, frog
GR: grape, great
PR: price, press
TR: train, tree
TW: twelve, twin
SLR: scrape, scratch
SPL: splash, split
SPR: spray, spring
SQU: square, squirt
STR: straw, street
THR: thread, thru

Form VM-20
SIGN LANGUAGE ALPHABET

Purpose: Spatial working memory that will go to long-term memory.

Materials: Pictures of sign language.

Method: The child will attempt to learn as many of the sign language letters as he can.

Levels 1 to 2: Show the child the hand position and see if he can imitate you. For these levels, just stay with copying your hand position.

Levels 3 to 5: Show the child one letter of the alphabet a day. Have him show it to you at his next therapy session. See how many letters of the alphabet he can learn.

The following pages are pictures of the sign language alphabet.

Form VM-20 (continued)
Sign Language Alphabet

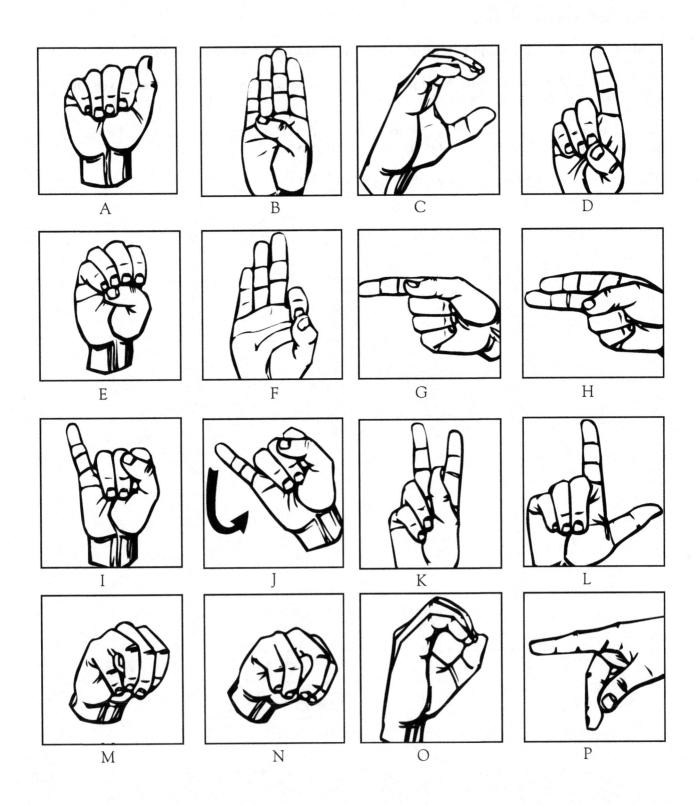

Form VM-20 (continued)
SIGN LANGUAGE ALPHABET

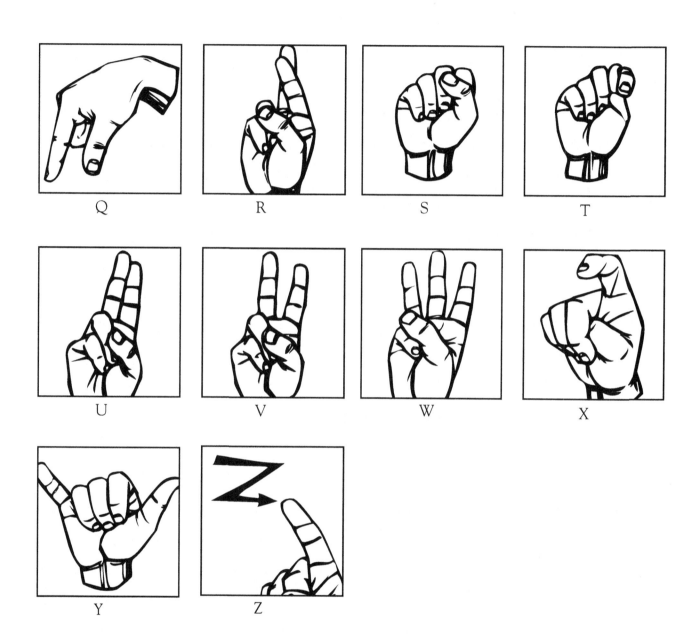

Q

R

S

T

U

V

W

X

Y

Z

VM-21
Word List/Two Second Span

Purpose: Working memory.

Materials: Sequences of words taken from the word list on these pages.

Method: The goal is to see how many words the child can remember in 2 seconds. For Levels 1 and 2, see how many letters a child can remember in 2 seconds.

Levels 1 to 2: Make a list of letters. Show the child the sequence of letters but only let him see it for 2 seconds.

Levels 3 to 5: Same as Levels 1 and 2, but use the words from the word list. The goal is six words in 2 seconds.

1	2	3	4	5	6
the	he	go	who	saw	big
a	I	see	an	home	where
is	they	then	their	soon	am
you	one	us	she	stand	ball
and	me	him	said	upon	live
we	about	by	did	first	four
that	had	was	boy	came	last
in	if	come	three	girl	color
not	some	get	down	house	away
for	up	or	work	find	red
at	her	two	put	because	friend
with	do	man	were	made	pretty
it	when	little	before	could	eat
on	so	has	just	book	want
can	my	them	long	look	year
will	very	how	here	mother	white
are	all	like	other	run	got
of	would	our	old	school	play
this	any	what	take	people	found
your	been	know	cat	night	left
as	out	make	again	into	men
but	there	which	give	say	bring
be	from	much	after	think	wish
have	day	his	many	back	black

VM-21 (continued)
WORD LIST/TWO SECOND SPAN

7	8	9	10	11	12
may	ran	ask	hat	off	fire
let	five	small	car	sister	ten
use	read	yellow	write	happy	order
these	over	show	try	once	part
right	such	goes	myself	didn't	early
present	way	clean	longer	set	fat
tell	too	buy	those	round	third
next	shall	thank	hold	dress	same
please	own	sleep	full	fall	love
leave	most	letter	carry	wash	hear
hand	sure	jump	eight	start	yesterday
more	thing	help	sing	always	eyes
why	only	fly	warm	anything	door
better	near	don't	sit	around	clothes
under	than	fast	dog	close	though
while	open	cold	ride	walk	o'clock
should	kind	today	hot	money	second
never	must	does	grow	turn	water
each	high	face	cut	might	town
best	far	green	seven	hard	took
another	both	every	woman	along	pair
seem	end	brown	funny	bed	now
tree	also	coat	yes	fine	keep
name	until	six	ate	sat	head
dear	call	gave	stop	hope	food

Form VM-22
CONSONANTS

Purpose: Short-term working memory.

Materials: Lists of words of no more than seven letters.

Method: Show the child the word for 4 seconds and then take it away. He is to tell you the locations of the consonants. For example, the word "system". He will tell you the positions of the consonants were 1, 2, 3, 4, 6. Try to work up to seven letter words.

Levels 1 to 2: Show the child the word and he tells you how many letters were in the word.

Levels 3 to 5: Use the method as discussed above with the consonants.

Form VM-23
VERB GENERATION

Purpose: Cerebellum and working memory.

Materials: A list of nouns. Have these on flash cards. Start with three and work up to seven.

Method: You flash the words to the child. Start with 4 seconds and work down to 2 seconds. He repeats the nouns and then tells you a verb that goes with them. For example:

apple = eat
car = ride
man = run

Level 2: Just have the child repeat the words.

Levels 3 to 5: The child must name the noun and tell you a verb that goes with it.

Form VM-24
GRID DOTS

Purpose: Visuospatial scratch pad.

Materials: Marker board or paper and pencil.

Method: Show the child your grid that has an X in one of the squares. He has a blank grid in front of him. Show him your grid and then take it away. Ask him questions like: If my X moved two squares to the right and down one, where would it end up? Put your X in your grid where you think it will end up. Example:

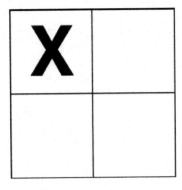

Only let him see your grid for 2 seconds.

Level 1: Only let the child copy where your X was. Use small grids like:

Form VM-24 (continued)
GRID DOTS

Level 2: Same as Level 1 but expand the grid.

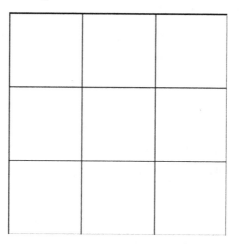

Levels 3 to 5: Now do as you were instructed in the example described in the Method section. Show him your grid. Take your grid away, and he is to put in his grid where your X will end up.

Form VM-25
WORD SHAPES A

Purpose: Central executive and working memory.

Materials: Marker board or paper and pencils.

Method: Assign letters to different shapes. For example:

short: a,c,e,i,m,n,o,r,s,u,v,w,x,z
tall: b,d,f,h,k,l,t
long: g,j,p,q,y

An example of letter spelling is as follows:
1. The word *read* would be: short, short, short, tall.
2. The word *pony* would be: long, short, short, long.
3. The word *yard* would be: long, short, short, tall.

Level 3:
1. Choose a category such as colors. Ask the child what color is spelled with three letters and is spelled short, short, tall. The answer is red.
2. What color is spelled with four letters and is tall, tall, short, short? The answer is blue.
3. Continue with other colors.

Level 4: Same as Level 3, but use other categories such as animals, food, drinks, etc.

Form VM-26
DUAL TASK

Purpose: Central executive.

Materials: Marker board or paper and pencils.

Method: Show the child a sequence of letters. For example: A C T Y O. Let him look at it for 4 seconds and then take it away. You will then ask him a series of questions that he must answer as true or false. For example, using the above sequence:

1. The letter T was between A and C: false
2. The Y followed the T: true
3. C is before the T but after the A: true

Level 3: Start with only four letters.

Levels 4 to 5: Start with five letters and work down from holding it 4 seconds to 2 seconds.

Form VM-27
WORD SHAPES B

Purpose: Central executive and working memory.

Materials: Marker board or pencil and paper.

Method: Assign letters to different shapes. For example: show the child the sequence of shapes and have him write what letters they were instead of shapes.

Levels 3 to 5: Follow the instructions under Method.

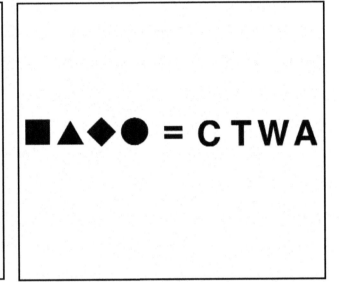

Chapter Eight

LATERALITY

Laterality is the internal awareness of the two sides of the body and of their difference. (LeFebrure, 1975)

Introduction

What is laterality? Why is it important and why are some of us left-handed and others right-handed? These are the questions that will be answered in this chapter. Anyone who has worked with children knows the term *laterality*, but why is it important to learning? The following are some definitions of laterality:

1. Kephart defines laterality as the internal awareness of the sides of the body and of knowing their differences (LeFebrure, 1975).
2. Piaget: Laterality is defined as the capacity to recognize through meaning, the right side and the left side of oneself, of someone opposite oneself, and of objects in space (LeFebrure, 1975).
3. Pieron tells us that laterality is the predominance of one or the other of two limbs (hand, eye) that determines sidedness (LeFebrure, 1975).

A more complete description would be that laterality is an emergence that comes from the operational organization of the two sides of the body, including the two brain hemispheres, and which would manifest itself as the completion of a process called "lateralization". The process of lateralization can be broken down into four major stages.

1. Monolateralization: from birth until approximately the 3rd month of life. At this stage, the two sides of the body, brain included, would function independently one from the other in such a way that the experiences lived by one side would not be sensed by the other.
2. Duolateralization: from approximately the 3rd month until the 12th month. The organism would then live the same experiences with both sides, either simultaneously or in rapid alternation for a complete integration.
3. Bilateralization: roughly from the 12th month until the 24th month. The child would reach this level of integration by setting active relations that will become more and more intricate between his paired limbs and within his basic biological, perceptual motor, and cognitive functions.
4. Integrated lateralization: from about the 42nd month. The proper organization of this stage would bring about the efficient use of the total body, brain included, stemming from the adequate assimilation of stimuli from the outside world, the adequate accommodation to these stimulations through proper reactions, and the adequate adaptation as a result of the equilibrium between past and present experiences and allowing for anticipation of the future (LeFebrure, 1975).

The following are some interesting facts concerning laterality:

1. Crossed dominance refers to the dominant eye being on one side of the body while the dominant hand is on the other side (Maples, 2002).
2. 10% more men than women are left-handed (*Health News*, 1992).
3. Handedness is established by 5 years of age (Maples, 2002).
4. Children under 7 years have developed both eye and hand preference.
5. Awareness of the left and right parts of one's body is usually established by 6 to 7 years; however, left/right discrimination for extra personal space is not established until 9 to 12 years (Tighe, 1968).
6. 71% of people are right-eye dominant (Maples, 2002).
7. Since Cro-Magnon man, humans have been overwhelmingly right-handed (90%) (Maples, 2002).
8. Delayed growth in the left hemisphere as a result of testosterone would account for greater frequency of left-handed males (Geschwind, 1982).
9. Between the ages of 6 and 7 years, the child's sense of right and left appears (Dequiros, 1979).
10. 58% of people are right-eyed dominant, 41.6% are left-eyed dominant, 87.1% are right-hand dominant and 12.9% are left-hand dominant.
11. 41.4% of people have crossed dominance between hand and eyes; 35% are right-handed and left-eyed.
12. Left-handedness runs in families (Rosenbaum, 2000).
13. Males are more likely to be left-handed (Rosenbaum, 2000).
14. In left-handed people, the right hemisphere controls speech and language in at least 30% of the cases (Rosenbaum, 2000).
15. Lefties die earlier.
16. A disproportionate number of left-handers are criminals.
17. Every US President for the last quarter century, with the exception of Jimmy Carter, was left-handed (Rosenbaum, 2000).
18. Of all the primates, only humans display a strong predisposition to right-handedness.

Explanations of handedness over the years have included position of the fetus, anatomical asymmetry, the body's center of gravity, heredity, eye dominance, hormonal imbalance, cerebral dominance, and social conditioning. It is a right-sided world. In Old English, the right hand was the strong hand, and the left was considered to be sinister (Dequiros, 1979). Even today, some cultures consider the left hand to be dirty (Maples, 2002). The English term for left derives from Celtic meaning "weak". The French feel it means awkward, and in Latin it means "sinister" and stands for evil. Ancient customs dictate that wedding rings should be worn on the left hand in belief that the precious metal will protect the body's weaker side from temptation (*Health News*, 1992).

The question that many have been trying to figure out for years is why some of us are left-handed and some right-handed. In her monograph, *Left, Right, Hand and Brain: The Right-Shift Theory*, Annett (1985) presents a genetic model that claims to explain the relationships between differences in hand performance, speech lateralization, and cognitive abilities on the basis of a hypothetical simple gene called the right-shift factor (rS) (Resch, 1997). Annett has proposed a theory of handedness and cerebral lateralization in which distribution of differences in skill between the hands is influenced by a single gene locus. Among individuals carrying the right shift (rs+) allele, the distribution is shifted in favor of right-handedness and left cerebral dominance for speech, more so in homozygotes (rs++ genotype) than in heterozygotes (rs+ genotype), while the distribution of those without the rr+ allele (rs-genotype) shows no overall biases in handedness or cerebral dominance. In a similar theory by McManus (1985), the focus is on hand preference rather than skills. McManus postulates a gene locus at which a dextral (D) allele predisposes towards right-hand preference, while a chance allele carries no directional bias so that hand preference is a matter of chance. In its simplest form, this model postulates that individuals homozygotic for the D allele (DD genotype) are all right-handed (Palmer, 1996).

These homozygotes for the C allele (cc genotype) are equally likely to be left or right-handed, while heterozygotes (DC genotype) have a .75 probability of being right-handed. This indicates that the chance of being right-handed is broken down as follows: 1/3 of individuals have 100% chance of being right-handed, 1/3 have a 50/50 chance of being right-handed, and the last 1/3 have a 75% chance of being right-handed. There is no left-hand gene (Palmer, 1996).

Research has shown that crossed eye dominance has not been caused by early developmental brain malfunc-

tion. Eye dominance has been reported to be established by 3 years of age (Maples, 2002).

A study that was published in the *Journal of Behavioral Optometry*, by W. C. Maples, OD, showed the following findings when considering school achievement and hand or eye dominance.

1. There was no significant difference in the total reading score between right- and left-handers between grades one through five.

2. There was a significant difference in the total reading score and reading comprehension scores between unidominant and crossed dominant children between grades one through five. The unidominant children scored higher. Unidominant means both eye and hand are the same dominance, for example, left eye and left hand.

3. Right-handed children, right-eye dominant children, and unidominant children did significantly better than their counterparts on the Visual Motor Integration Test (VMI).

4. Right-eye dominant children and unidominant children did significantly better on the Wold Sentence Copy Test than their counterparts (Maples, 2002).

Laterality Tips

1. Make sure you are not trying to make the child do something that he is not mature enough to do. For example, you can't make a 5-year-old child understand the relationships between an external object's right/left orientation and his own.

2. Before you attempt reversal training, the child needs a good understanding of his own right and left.

References

Annett, M. (1989). The disadvantages of dextrality for intelligence. *British Journal of Psychology, 80*, 213-226.

Dequiros, J. B. (1979). *Neuropsychological fundamentals in learning disabilities*. Novato, CA: Academic Therapy Publications.

Geschwind, N. (1982). Left handedness: Association with immune disease, migraine and developmental learning disorder. *Psychology, 79*, 5097-5100.

Lane, K. A. (1995). Parents' satisfaction with vision therapy. *Journal of Behavioral Optometry, 6*(6), 151-153.

LeFebrure, J. J. (1975). Laterality: Multisensorial stimulation. *Journal of Optometric Development, 5*(2), 7-15.

Maples, W. C. (2002). Handedness, eyedness, hand-eye dominance & academic performance. *Journal of Behavioral Optometry, 13*(4), 87-90.

McMonnies, C. W. (1992). Reversals and left/right confusion. *Journal of Behavioral Optometry, 3*(2), 31-34.

Palmer, R. (1996). Predicting reading ability from handedness measures. *British Journal of Psychology, 87*(4), 609-620.

Resch, F. (1997). Testing the hypothesis of the relationships between laterality and ability according to Annet's right-shift theory: Findings in an epidemiological sample of young adults. *British Journal of Psychology, 88*(4), 621-635.

Rosenbaum, D. B. (2000). On left-handedness, its causes and costs. *The New York Times.* May 16, 2000.

The left-handed riddle. (1992). *Health News, 10*(2), 84.

Tighe, T. J. (1968). Perceptual learning in the discrimination processes of children: An analysis of five variables in perceptual pretraining. *American Psychological Association, 77,* 125-133.

Form L-I
HEAD ROLL

Purpose: Laterality.

Materials: Metronome for Level 2.

Method: Lie the child down on his back, legs together, arms at his side. Have the child look at an object on the ceiling directly above his head. Children under 6 are too young to have a good understanding of their right and left. If the child is younger than 6, help him by showing him which direction is right and which is left throughout this activity.

Observations: Make sure the child leads with his eyes as he turns his head.

Level 1: At your command, he is to turn his head to the right and look at an object on his right. Next, at your command, he turns his head back to the object on the ceiling, and finally, on command, to an object on his left. For example, you call out right and he turns his head to the right and then back to look at an object on the ceiling.

Level 2: Set the metronome to about 40 beats per minute. At each beat, he is to change head position, first to the right then back to the ceiling and finally to the left. He is to call out "right" or "left" as he turns his head. He continues until you tell him to stop. For example, he will say "right", "ceiling", "left", "ceiling", "right", "ceiling", etc.

Form L-2
BODY ROLL

Purpose: Laterality.

Materials: None.

Method: Child lies on his back with his legs together and arms at his side.

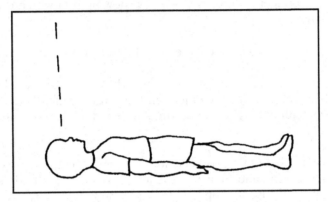

Observations: Make sure he leads with his eyes.

Level 1:
1. At your command, he is to push off with his left arm and roll completely to the right until he is again looking straight up at the ceiling. Tell him he is rolling right. You will have to show him which of his hands are right or left.

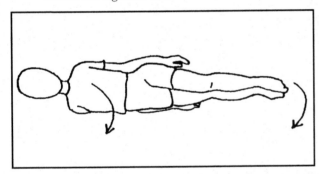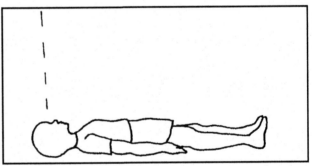

2. Do the same as #1, but have him roll to the left as he pushes off with his right arm. Tell him he is rolling left.

Level 2:
1. When you clap once, have him push off with his left arm and roll completely to his right until he is again looking straight up at the ceiling. He is to call out "right" as he rolls right. When you clap twice, he rolls to his left by pushing off with his right arm. He is to call out "left" as he rolls left. Vary your clapping. For example, you may clap for him to go right two times in a row.

Form L-2 (continued)
BODY ROLL

Level 3: Same as Level 2, but tell him to remember the sequence of claps you give him and roll in the proper sequence. For example, clap..........clap clap.........clap would be roll right, roll left, roll right. Clap, clap............clap clap would be roll left, roll left. Work up to five commands in a roll.

Form L-3
MAZE GAME

Purpose: Laterality.

Materials: Marker board.

Method: For Level 3, draw objects on the marker board. Make them various sizes and various distances from each other. For example:

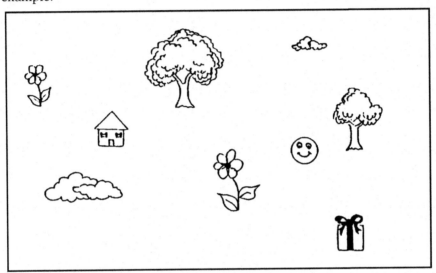

On each level, the child must get through the maze without hitting an object.

Level 2:
1. Have the child stand at one end of the room. Scatter chairs or other objects around the room. The child closes his eyes and starts to walk through the maze. You help him by calling out "left" or "right" as he nears an obstacle.
2. Repeat #1, but see if he can remember where the obstacles are. Don't help him by calling out "left" or "right".

Level 3:
1. Child puts his marker at one end of the board. He closes his eyes and tries to get through the maze without hitting any of the objects. You help him by calling out "up", "down", "left" or "right" as he gets near an object.
2. Do both in vertical and horizontal directions. Have him alternate hands.
3. Reduce the number of targets on the board and see if he can remember and get through the maze without you calling out directions.

Levels 4-5:
1. Same as Level 2 #1 and 2, but the child is to go in the opposite direction from the one you call. For example, if you tell him to go "left", he will have to go right to keep from hitting the target. If you say go "up", he will have to go down.

Form L-4
FLASHLIGHT WALKING

Purpose: Laterality.

Materials: Two flashlights.

Method: The child holds a flashlight in each hand.

Levels 3 to 4: The child is instructed to point the flashlight to either the foot on the same side as his hand holding the flashlight, or the opposite foot as he walks slowly forward. He is to call out the name of the foot that makes the forward movement with the flashlight pointing at it. For example, "left foot". He is then to call out the hand holding the flashlight that is pointing to the forward foot. For example, "left hand". If he was pointing the flashlights to the opposite feet, an example of a sequence might be: "left foot" "right hand", "right foot" "left hand", etc.

Form L-5
WALKING PROCEDURE

Purpose: Laterality.

Materials: Metronome.

Method: Have the child do the following activities.

Level 2: As the child walks, he calls out, "right hand up", "right leg up", "right hand down", "right leg down". Each time the child says what is to be moved and calls it out as he moves those limbs. He alternates between right and left sides as he walks a distance of 10 to 12 feet.

Level 3:
1. As the child walks, he picks up his leg, calling it up. For example, left leg up. Then he lifts up his arm on his other side, calling it up. For example, right arm up. He then puts that arm down first, calling it down, then puts the leg down, taking a step and calling it down at the same time.
2. When the child walks forward, have him call each arm as it moves up and down. For example, "right arm up", "right arm down", "left arm up", "left arm down". When he starts to walk backward, have him call out which leg is moving up and down.
3. Same as #1, but on this procedure, set the metronome at 40 beats per minute. Have the child say only one word per beat. For example, on beat one the child would say "right", on beat two, he would say "hand", beat three would be "up". This is a very slow cadence, and for some children it is difficult to stay with the beat.

Levels 4 to 5: Set the metronome to 40 beats per minute. As the child walks forward, he is to say three words per beat. For example, on the first beat, "right arm up", on the second beat "left leg up", on the third beat "left leg down", etc. For children who are unaccustomed to doing things quickly, it may be very difficult for them to say all three words to one beat and move as they say it.

Form L-6
NUMBERED CIRCLES ON MARKER BOARD

Purpose: Laterality.

Materials: Marker board, metronome.

Method: The numbers 1 to 5 are placed randomly on the marker board (as the child becomes good at this the numbers can be increased). The child stands in front of the board and circles each number three times. After the third time, he draws a line from number 1 to number 2, circles that three times, and then proceeds to each succeeding number.

Level 1: Have the child circle each number three times. Have him do it first with his right hand and then with his left.

Level 2:
1. Have the child circle all the numbers clockwise or counterclockwise. You may need to show him what is clockwise or counterclockwise.
2. Have the child circle all even numbers clockwise and all odd numbers counterclockwise.

Levels 3 to 5:
1. Have the child circle all the numbers clockwise or counterclockwise. Numbers are circled to the beat of the metronome, starting at the top of the circle on the first beat and the bottom of the circle on the second beat.
2. Use any combination and any number of circles. Letters can be used and have the child spell out words.

Form L-7
ANGELS IN THE SNOW

Purpose: Laterality.

Materials: Marsden ball, metronome.

Method: Child lies on his back on the floor with arms along the side of his body and his heels touching. As you touch or call out one or more of his limbs, he moves them out and away from his body.

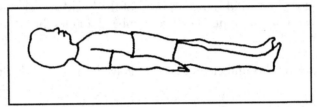

Observations: Limbs are not to move off the floor. He is to drag them across the floor. Limbs are to reach the end positions at the same time. End position for legs is spread out as far as possible.

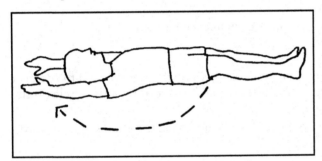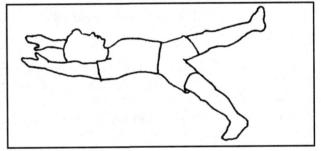

Level 1:
1. Touch the arm or leg you want him to move. He calls out what he is doing and moves the limb.
2. Repeat #1, but point to the limb to be moved. Don't touch it.

Level 2: Child is to move two limbs so that they arrive at the extreme outward position at the same time. For example, both arms over his head, or right arm and right leg or right arm and left leg.

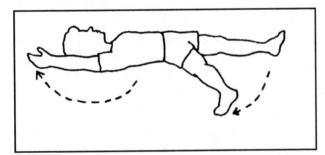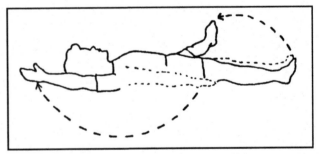

Level 3:
1. Set metronome at about 40 beats per minute. Use any arm and leg combination. The limbs are to be moved by a certain number of beats, usually starting with four. They are both to arrive at their extreme position at the end of four beats and start their return and arrive at their original position by the end of another four beats.
2. Increase to eight beats.

Form L-7 (continued)
ANGELS IN THE SNOW

Level 4:

1. With this activity, you will use a Marsden ball. This is a ball about the size of a tennis ball, hanging from the ceiling about 3 feet over the child's chest. The child is to lie under the Marsden ball. Swing the ball in a head to foot direction. Tell the child that when the ball is up toward his head, his right arm and right leg will be out and when it is at this feet, his left arm and left leg will be out and his right arm and right leg will be back at the starting position.

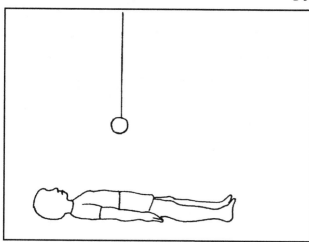 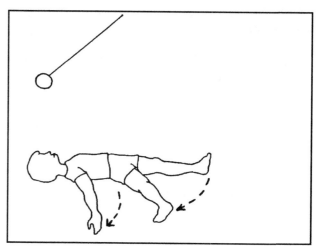

2. Vary the direction of ball and limbs to be moved. For example, swing the ball left to right. When it is at his right, both arms go over his head. When it is at his left, both legs go out and the arms go back to his side.

Level 5: Set metronome to about 40 beats per minute. Use any leg and arm combination. The limbs are to be moved to a certain number of beats. They are to arrive at their extreme positions at the end of the required number of beats, and return to their original position at the required number of beats. Vary the number of beats per limb. For example, arms over the head in four beats and legs out in eight beats. Use any limb and beat combination.

Form L-8
CODING ON MARKER BOARD

Purpose: Laterality.

Materials: Marker board.

Method: Draw an outline of back and shoulder area with nine circles on it on the marker board at the child's own height. When you touch one of the spots on his back, he is to point to the corresponding spot on the drawing on the board.

Level 2: Touch each of the nine indicated spots on his back until he can locate each one accurately on the marker board before him.

Level 3: Tap a pattern from one spot to another rhythmically, starting with two locations and building up to three or more. Repeat in irregular rhythms. He duplicates the pattern on the board.

Levels 4 to 5: Trace a line from one dot to the next on his back. Have him duplicate it on the board. He must draw in the same direction.

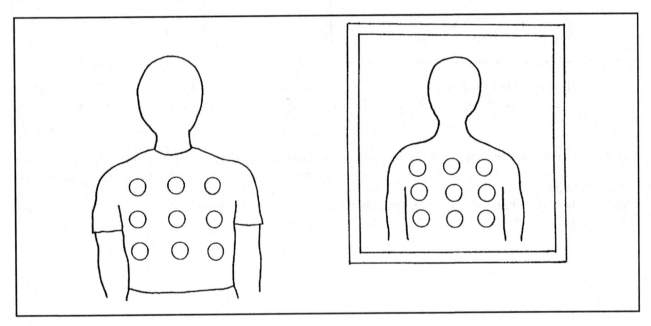

Form L-9
TACTILE REINFORCEMENT

Purpose: Laterality.

Materials: Plastic letters in Level 3.

Method: The child will follow your directions with his eyes closed.

Level 2:
1. The child has his eyes closed. You touch a part of his body. The child is to say what part and on what side. For example, right side of face.
2. The child has his eyes closed and his hands on the table. Touch one of his fingers and have him move it. Touch two fingers simultaneously and have him move them.

Level 3:
1. The child has his eyes closed with his hands in a neutral position. For example, directly in front of him on a table. You move his hands to a new position for 2 seconds and then back to the neutral position. The child must open his eyes and move his hands to the position you had them. You can use one or both of his hands for this activity.
2. The child has his eyes closed. Put various objects or letters in his hand. Have him tell you what these are with his eyes closed.

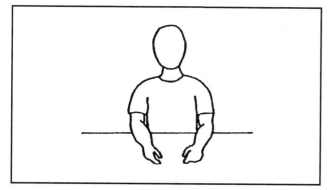 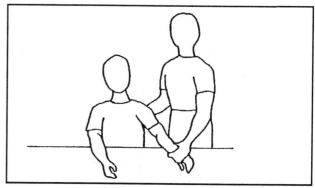

Levels 4 to 5: The child has his eyes closed. Draw a simple design on the back of his hand and have him open his eyes and draw it on the board.

Form L-10
THE CLOCK GAME

Purpose: Laterality.

Materials: Marker board.

Method: On the marker board, place eight points equally spaced around the circumference of a circle approximately 18 inches in diameter. For example:

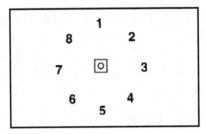

The points should be arranged so that one and five determine a vertical axis, points seven and three determine a horizontal axis, and points six and two, eight and four determine two diagonal axes. In the center is a box with an O in the center. The box is the goal for all movement terminating in the center of the circle. In all activities the child should move both hands simultaneously and they should arrive at their respective goals at the same time. Have the child start with each hand on the starting number and move to the stop number. The child should tell you the direction each of his hands will move before he moves it. For example, in Level 2, he will say, "I will move my left hand left and my right hand right."

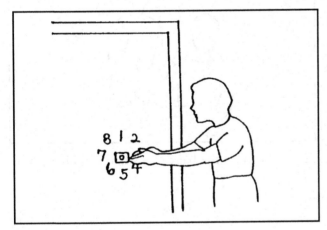
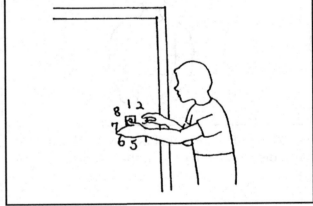

Level 2:
1. Toward the Center. In this activity, the child is to start with his two hands on the circumference of the circle and is asked to bring them both toward the center. Use the following order.

Left Hand		**Right Hand**	
Start	*Stop*	*Start*	*Stop*
7	0	3	0
1	0	5	0
5	0	1	0
8	0	4	0
6	0	2	0

Form L-10 (continued)
THE CLOCK GAME

2. Opposed Movement Away from Center

Left Hand		Right Hand	
Start	*Stop*	*Start*	*Stop*
0	7	0	3
0	1	0	5
0	5	0	1
0	8	0	4
0	6	0	2

3. Parallel Movement

Left Hand		Right Hand	
Start	*Stop*	*Start*	*Stop*
7	0	0	3
0	7	3	0
1	0	0	5
0	1	5	0
5	0	0	1
0	5	1	0
8	0	0	4
0	8	4	0
6	0	0	2
0	6	2	0

Form L-10 (continued)
THE CLOCK GAME

Level 3:
1. Movement with Cross Meridians, Movement Toward Center

Left Hand		Right Hand	
Start	*Stop*	*Start*	*Stop*
7	0	1	0
7	0	5	0
1	0	3	0
5	0	3	0
8	0	1	0
8	0	3	0
8	0	5	0
6	0	1	0
6	0	3	0
6	0	5	0
8	0	2	0
6	0	4	0
7	0	2	0
7	0	4	0
1	0	2	0
1	0	4	0
5	0	2	0
5	0	4	0

2. Movement Away From Center

Left Hand		Right Hand	
Start	*Stop*	*Start*	*Stop*
0	7	0	2
0	7	0	5
0	1	0	3
0	5	0	3
0	8	0	1
0	8	0	3
0	8	0	5
0	6	0	1
0	6	0	3
0	6	0	5
0	8	0	2
0	6	0	4
0	7	0	2
0	7	0	4
0	1	0	2
0	1	0	4
0	5	0	2
0	5	0	4

Form L-10 (continued)
THE CLOCK GAME

Levels 4 to 5:

1. Cross Movement – Cross Meridian, Movement Left to Right

Left Hand		Right Hand	
Start	*Stop*	*Start*	*Stop*
7	0	0	1
7	0	0	5
7	0	0	2
7	0	0	4
8	0	0	3
8	0	0	5
8	0	0	1
8	0	0	2
6	0	0	3
6	0	0	1
6	0	0	4
6	0	0	0

2. Movement to Left, Cross Movement

Left Hand		Right Hand	
Start	*Stop*	*Start*	*Stop*
0	7	1	0
0	7	5	0
0	7	2	0
0	7	4	0
0	8	3	0
0	8	5	0
0	8	1	0
0	8	2	0
0	6	3	0
0	6	1	0
0	6	4	0
0	6	5	0

Form L-11
MIDLINE TRAINING

Purpose: Laterality.

Materials: Penlight.

Method: Follow the directions in each section. Explain what a midline is and show the child both his midline and your midline.

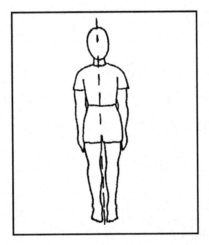

Level 1: Have the child hold his arms straight out in front of him. Have him move his arms out all the way to his sides and back to the starting point. Each time his arms move out, he is to say "out". Each time his arms move in, he is to say "in". Repeat with his eyes closed.

Level 2: Have him hold his right arm pointing to the right as he faces straight ahead. Have him move his arms towards his midline and call out "out-in" as he does it. Have him stop at his midline, continue from the midline calling out "in-out" until his right arm is pointing all the way to his left. Repeat this with his left arm going from left to right. Do this with his eyes open and closed.

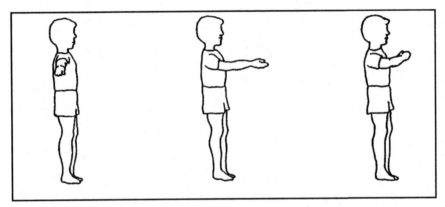

Form L-11 (continued)
MIDLINE TRAINING

Level 3:

1. Have him hold his right arm pointing to the right as he faces straight ahead. Have him move his arm towards his midline and call out "right to left" and stop at his midline. As he continues from midline, he again calls out "left". Do the same thing with his arm going from left to right.

2. Repeat #1, but with his right arm pointing all the way to the left and going from left to right and have him call out "left to right". Do the same with his left arm pointing to the right and going from right to left.

3. Do both #1 and 2 again, but don't stop at midline. Make a continuous motion going from either right to left or left to right. Do with eyes open and closed.

Levels 4 to 5: Darken the room and have the child seated in a chair. Stand across the room with a penlight. Start on his right side and have him call out "right to left" as it approaches his midline and again "right to left" as it crosses his midline. Do the same thing starting on his left side.

Form L-12
RECIPROCAL MOVEMENTS

Purpose: Laterality.

Materials: None.

Method: The child is to imitate your movements.

Level 1:
1. Have the child stand in front of you with his hands in front of him at chest level. Have him open one of his hands while he closes the other. This can also be done to a metronome.
2. With his arms out at his side, at shoulder level, have him move one arm up while the other moves down.
3. Have him move one arm up and the leg on the opposite side out.

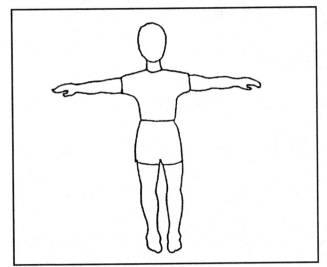 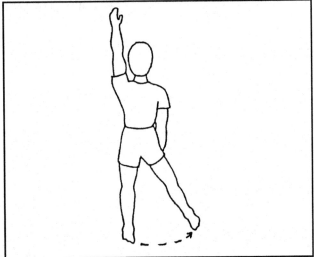

Level 2:
1. Stand in front of the child with your arms out at the side at shoulder level and have him move the same side as you do. For example, you move your right arm up and he moves his left arm up.
2. Stand in front of the child. Have him move the same limb as you, as if he were facing in your direction. For example, you move your left arm up, he moves his left arm up.

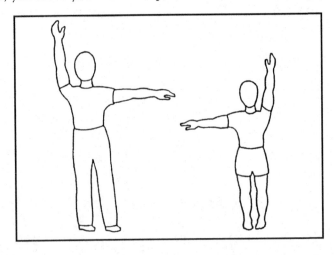

Form L-12 (continued)
RECIPROCAL MOVEMENTS

Level 3: Stand in front of the child with both of your arms out at the side at shoulder level. Have him move the same limb as you as he would if he was facing in your direction. For example, you move your right arm up, he moves his right arm down, you move your arm in towards your body, he moves his out.

Levels 4 to 5: Stand next to the child with both arms out at the side at shoulder level. The child must imitate in reverse with one side of his body these movements imposed by you on the other side of his body. For example, you move your right arm up as he moves his left arm down. Start next to the child. Move later to face him.

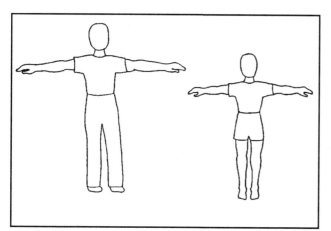
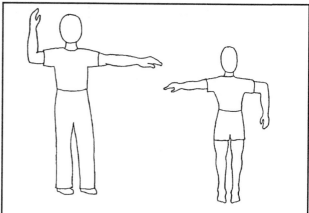

Form L-13
Tic-Tac-Toe

Purpose: Laterality.

Materials: Marker board.

Method: You will play tic-tac-toe with the child using the marker board.

Level 2:
1. The child must call out the square he wants to put his X in. For example, "top left".

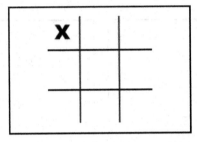

2. He puts his X in the square, you then put your O in the square you want.

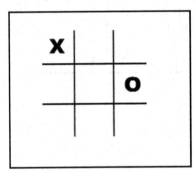

3. The child only gets one chance at naming the correct square. If he calls out "top right", that's the square the X goes in.

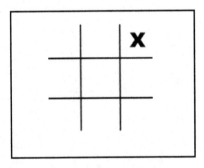

Levels 3 to 5: Child must call out the square he wants to put his X in. For example, "top left". For this activity, he does not mark it on the board. He must remember where he put the X. You can put your Os on the board, but he must remember where he put his Xs.

Form L-14
Xs Procedure

Purpose: Laterality.

Materials: Marker board, metronome.

Method: Place seven Xs on the marker board with the center X at nose height. The side Xs are 12 to 18 inches from the center X (the distance is dependent on the child's size). Two other Xs are placed directly above and directly below the side Xs. Have the child hold a piece of chalk in each hand.

```
   X                    X

   X          X         X

   X                    X
```

The child starts by placing the chalk on the Xs you tell him and he follows your directions as to what directions you want him to move each hand. Each hand always goes from the starting X to the designated X and then back to the starting X.

Level 2:
1. The right hand marker is placed on the right X and the left hand marker on the left X. Tell the child to look at the center X. Then move each marker to the center X and back to the starting place, one at a time, as he calls out which hand he is going to move.
2. Tell him to move his right hand first then his left hand and then both hands saying "right", "left", "both" as he does it. This results in his right hand going to the center and his left hand going to the center and then both hands going back to their starting places.
3. Another variation of this is "right, both, left". When he says "right" the right hand goes from right to center; on "both" the left hand goes from left to center and the right hand from center to right; and on "left" the left hand goes from center to left.

Levels 3 to 5:
1. The child is instructed to move his marker from any X to any other X. For example, the right hand can go from the right X to the top right X while the left hand goes from the left side X to the bottom left X. For example, a command of right, left, both would be moving the right marker to the top right X, moving the left marker to the lower left X, and moving both hands back to the starting points.
2. Use the metronome. He does one movement to each beat.
3. Increase the directions to four then five. For example, four directions can be "right, both, left, both".
4. Place the Xs in different positions. The three horizontal Xs remain in the same position, but the vertical Xs are changed.

Form L-15
ARROWS ON BOARD

Purpose: Laterality.

Materials: Marker board, metronome.

Method: Draw four arrows on the board. Draw one up, one down, one to the right, and one to the left. The child is to stand about 10 feet in front of them. For example:

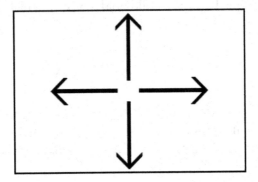

Each time he hears the metronome, he moves his hands to another arrow and calls out the direction it is pointing. Work clockwise or counterclockwise.

Level 1: Child stands in front of the arrows. Each time he hears the metronome, he holds his hands together and points them in the direction the arrows are pointing and calls out the direction. Start with the top arrow and work clockwise or counter clockwise. For example:

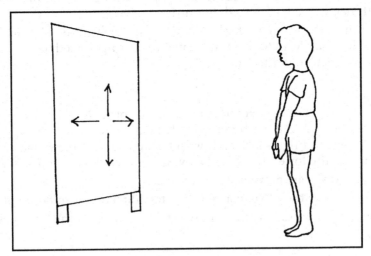

Levels 2 to 3: This time he points with both hands held together and when the arrows are pointing up or down and with his right hand for the right arrow and his left hand for the left arrow.

Form L-15 (continued)
ARROWS ON BOARD

Levels 4 to 5:

1. Add four more arrows. For example:

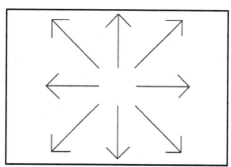

   Have the child just use one hand and call out the directions of the arrows at the beat of the metronome. For example, top, top right, right, bottom right, bottom, bottom left, left, top left.

2. Vary this by having him point with both hands held together for the top and bottom arrows and the right hand for the right arrows and the left hand for the left arrows.

Form L-16
VERTICAL LINES

Purpose: Laterality.

Materials: Visual motor activity sheet, metronome.

Method: The child is seated at a table with you next to him. He is to hold the activity sheet at normal reading distance. At the beat of the metronome, he calls out the position of the vertical line to the horizontal line. For example, the top row going left to right would be right up, middle down, right down, left up.

Levels 3 to 5:
1. Have him do each row in a left to right direction, calling out the positions.
2. Have him go in a vertical direction.
3. Without the metronome, time him in both the horizontal and vertical directions. Record his speed.

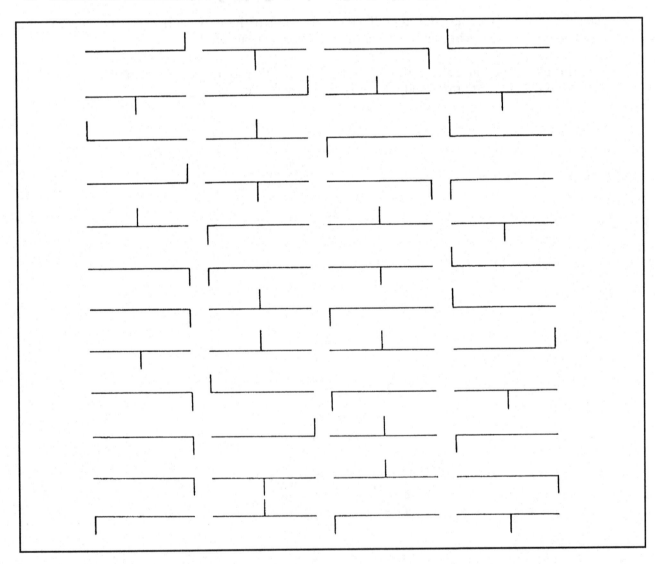

Form L-17
BODY AWARENESS

Purpose: Laterality.

Materials: None.

Method: Have the child do the following.

Levels 1 to 2: Have the child sit on the floor, knees bent, feet flat on the floor. Tell him to do the following.
1. Put your left hand on your right toe.
2. Clap your hands twice.
3. Put your left hand on your left toe.
4. Put your elbows together.
5. Touch your heels.
6. Touch your eyes.
7. Put your feet apart.
8. Touch one elbow.
9. Touch two elbows.
10. Draw a square in the air.
11. Clap one time.
12. Clasp your hands behind your neck.
13. Touch one shoulder.
14. Put your knees together.
15. Touch your right knee with your left hand.
16. Touch your left knee with your right hand.
17. Place your palms together.
18. Clap your hands twice.
19. Touch one knee and one foot.
20. Put your hands on your head.
21. Touch your nose.
22. Touch your toes with your arms crossed.
23. Touch your nose with one hand, your knee with the other.
24. Put your right hand on your left knee.
25. Cross your arms in front of your chest.
26. Put your right hand over your left eye.
27. Cross your arms in front of your chest.
28. Put your left hand on your right knee.
29. Put your right hand on your left hip.
30. Cross your arms in front of your chest.
31. Put your left hand on your right hip.

Form L-17 (continued)
BODY AWARENESS

32. Cross your arms in front of your chest.
33. Put your left hand on your right foot.
34. Cross your arms in front of your chest.
35. Put your right hand on your left foot.
36. Cross your right arm in front of your chest.
37. Put your left hand on your right ear.
38. Cross your arms in front of your chest.
39. Put your right hand on your left ear.
40. Cross your arms in front of your chest.

Form L-18
LATERALITY CODING

Purpose: Laterality.

Materials: Marker board or paper, Laterality Coding Chart.

Method: The following symbols are used in this activity:

b = hand	d = foot
lb = left hand	bl = right hand
ld = left foot	dl = right foot
db = both hands	qp = both feet
dbl = right foot and right hand	
ldb = left foot and left hand	

Use the Laterality Coding Chart and as you point to each symbol, the child will either raise his hand or stomp the appropriate foot. He should also call out which hand or foot he is using. For example, left foot, right hand, etc.

Levels 3 to 5: Go through the chart in a left to right direction. Then go through the chart in a top to bottom direction.

db	lb	dl	qp
dbl	ldb	lb	ldb
d	b	dbl	dl
bl	dl	qp	ldb
ld	dl	db	dbl

Form L-19
DIRECTIONAL "U" SACCADES

Purpose: Directionality.

Materials: Directional "U" worksheet.

Method: Set the metronome at 60 beats per minute (slower or faster if desired). The child stands 20 feet away from the worksheet, which is hung on the wall.

Level 1: Tell the child to clasp his hands together and extend them in front of himself. To each beat of the metronome, he is to move his hands in the direction of the opening in each "U". Do each line in a left to right manner.

Levels 2 to 5:
1. Tell the child to clasp his hands together and extend them in front of himself. To each beat of the metronome, he is to move his hands in the direction of the opening of each "U" and call out the directions (right, left, up or down). Do each line in a left to right manner.
2. Repeat #1, going down the vertical columns from top to bottom.
3. Without the metronome and without using his hands, see how fast he can do both the horizontal and vertical rows and call out the direction of each opening.

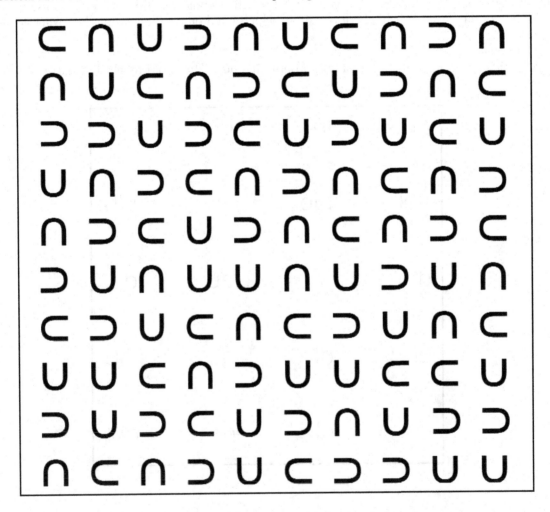

Form L-20
Directional Arrows

Purpose: Directionality.

Materials: Metronome, Directional Arrows form below.

Method: The child is seated at a table with you sitting next to him. Have him hold the worksheet below at normal reading distance.

Level 2:
1. At the beat of the metronome, the child is to name the direction of each arrow. Start on the horizontal line and move in a left to right sequence.
2. Same as #1, but go down the vertical lines from top to bottom.
3. Without the metronome, time him and see how fast he can do the horizontal and vertical lines.

Levels 3 to 5: At the beat of the metronome, the child is to walk in a heel to toe manner on the walking rail. As he walks, have him call out the direction of the arrows. Go in both the horizontal direction and the vertical direction.

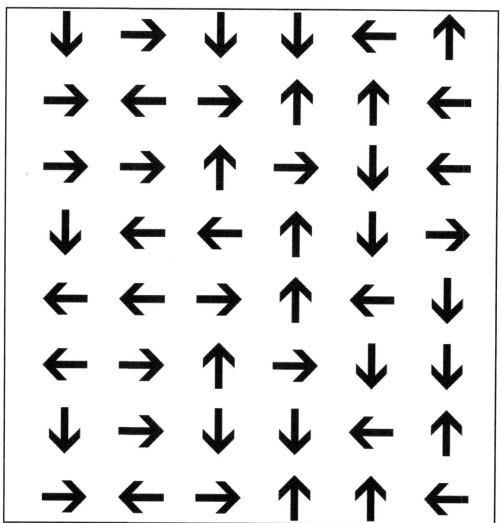

Chapter Nine

REVERSALS

The assumption that children will outgrow reversals is not valid.

(McMonnies, 1992)

There are several things that you should know about reversals.

1. It is normal to reverse, but it is to a greater extent with dyslexics (McMonnies, 1992).

2. There are twice as many reversals in the horizontal compared to the vertical plane. There is a 2:1 ratio bias towards right to left reversals as opposed to left to right due to a failure of children to establish stable left to right habits of visual scanning (Fischer, 1971).

3. The ability of a young child to look at an object and know that it is still the same object even if it is upside down is called *object constancy*. Some believe that the establishment of object constancy is the cause of reversal confusions with letters b, d, p, and q and the sequence order of letters in words.

4. Poor readers make more reversals than good readers (Harman, 1982).

5. Mirror reading and writing are more common in left handers. We don't know why (Heilman, 1980).

6. There are indications that young children have a tendency to begin their inspection of a pattern from the right rather than the left, differing in this regard from older children and adults who begin from the left (McMonnies, 1992).

7. The incidence of b/d confusion in dyslexics is at least 65%. The reversal errors said to be characteristic of dyslexics account for 20 to 25% of their reading problems.

8. In dyslexics, 30% of 12 to 14-year-olds and 12% of 15 to 81-year-olds still have b/d confusion.

9. If a child is older than 7 to 8 and still reverses, it could be an indication of reading difficulties (Kaufman, 1980).

10. There is a correlation of .49 between reversal and reading achievement (Kaufman, 1980).

11. The assumption that children always grow out of their reversals is not valid (McMonnies, 1992).

12. Reversals constitute approximately 45% of all errors of 4-year-olds, drops to about 23% of all 5-year-olds, and drops to about 5% of all 7-year-olds (Moyer, 1977).

Orientation processes low salience on a hierarchy of qualities or attributes that a child can respond to when performing match to sample tests. It has been reported that children 3 to 8 years of age respond to the contour of forms before responding to any details drawn on them. Orientation proved to be the discriminative cue of least information. Three to 5-year-olds see differences in orientation but do not consider them when judging sameness.

Orientation appears to be of little value to young children (Kaufman, 1980).

Reversals have been found in some brain injury cases, especially those affecting parietal and occipital regions (Frith, 1971).

The one area that you will be asked about more often than anything else is reversals. Parents seem to have a fear that if their child reverses letters or words then he is dyslexic. Several months ago, I had a parent who came into my office concerned that her son was reversing. Her son was 5 years old. We may laugh at this since he was only 5 years old, but the parent had a real concern. The first thing we need to do is to tell the parents what to expect with reversals by the age of the child. Children need a mental age of 5½ to 6½ to overcome "up-down" (vertical) reversals and 7½ for "left-right" (horizontal) reversals (Harman, 1982). By the end of second grade, reversals occur only among the poorest readers (Fischer, 1971). By the age of 9 or 10 years, children are said to code spatial location in adult-like fashion, enabling them to understand how the relationships among objects would appear at various angles (Wallace, 2001). The fact of the matter is that all children will reverse. It is only when it's excessive or persists past second grade that it is a concern. Even adults will reverse at times. It is up to us to determine if a child is having a learning problem due to their reversals and then help the child to overcome them. My rule of thumb is to ask the parent if the child reverses and if so, how often. I then ask if he is having difficulty learning in school. If the child is not having any learning problems and only reverses infrequently, I don't worry about it; however, if the child seems to reverse a lot and is having difficulty learning to read, then remedial measures need to be taken.

Reversals are of two kinds. The first group is *kinetic* reversals. These are reversals caused by writing or printing in which the child has to move his hand to form a stroke sequence. The second group is *static*, in which there is no movement by the child and he is confused on the proper orientation of the letter or letter sequences in a word as he reads. The first area we will discuss will be static reversals.

Static Reversals

One of the oldest theories is Orton's Cerebral Dominance Theory and was proposed in 1925 by Orton. He used the term *stephosymbolia,* or twisted symbols, to describe errors of this sort and considered them to be an important cause of reading disabilities. According to Orton, reversal errors were due to a conflict between mirror image representations of a symbol in the right and left hemisphere of the brain. When neither hemisphere was dominant, the two conflicting mirror images created perceptual confusion. Reversals, therefore, were indicative of neurological malfunction. Currently, Orton's conceptualizations regarding cerebral dominance have little credibility among neurologists. The concept of hemispheric dominance has been supplemented in modern neurological theory by the concept of hemisphere specialization—the idea that each hemisphere performs certain functions more efficiently than the other (Moyer, 1977). Another theory is that children who persistently fail to acquire a preference for the given spatial orientation of letters as rapidly as normal readers are deficient in one or several of these areas: attention, learning, and memory (Frith, 1971). Many young children do not consider the orientation of a letter to be important. I call this 3D – 2D confusion. The child has been raised in a three-dimensional world. All the objects that he has been exposed to did not change identification due to their orientation. A cup was a cup no matter which way the handle was pointing. It is only when the child gets into school and is faced with two-dimensional print that he becomes confused. For the first time in his life, he is faced with an identification problem due to spatial awareness. He finds that the letter "b" changes completely when it is faced the other way and becomes "d" or the word "was" changes when it is "saw". These children are not suffering from a neurological impairment, they are simply confusing two similar graphic displays. It has been shown that orientation has the lowest weight of value for young children in form recognition. Three to 5-year-olds may actually see the difference, but do not consider it important when judging sameness (Harman, 1982). Young children must have a good understanding of their own body imagery as a necessary condition for discrimination of mirror images. If a child can't differentiate between left and right, he can't be expected to differentiate between b and d (Simner, 1984).

What happens to children who reverse letters and words? They tend to reverse the same letters and words consistently. For example, the letters classically reversed by children said to be dyslexic are p, q, b, d, u and n; the words are was, saw, no, on, pot, top, and of and for and stop for spot. However, there is something interesting about these letters and words. They are not randomly chosen. Rather they seem to be chosen because they make sense when reversed. They are not suffering from a brain malfunction but are suffering from an inability to spatially discriminate letters, while for word reversals, it is usually due to poor reading skills. They are reading one word at a time and not for comprehension (Harman, 1982). For example, does the child really mean to reverse the word "saw" in the sentence? I saw a monkey, and say I was a monkey. The child reversed saw because he was scanning the words from right to left and was only reading one word at a time and not for reading comprehension.

Another theory that should be discussed is that because the "b" type letters and numbers in the English alphanumeric series exceed the "d" type of letters and numbers by a ratio of 2 to 1, and since "e" is the most frequently used letter of the alphabet, it can be assumed that a left to right bias may be formed that will cause children to reverse left facing letters and numbers more often than right facing letters and numbers. If a child is confused and doesn't know which way to print it, he has better odds if he faces it in the right instead of left direction (Simner, 1984).

It appears that the most likely cause of static reversals is poor reading skills when dealing with word reversals and immature spatial and discrimination abilities when dealing with static letter and number reversals.

Kinetic Reversals

The next category of reversals deals with kinetic reversals. These are printing and writing reversals (Figure 9-1).

Mirror reading and mirror writing appear to be more common in three populations: the left handed, retarded and dyslexic children. In their motor skills, left handers tend to be more ambidextrous than are right-handers. Moreover, it appears that the cerebral organization of left-handers is less asymmetrical than that of right-handers. Therefore, it would be more likely to confuse right and left on themselves and in space. Because some left-handers may have less of an asymmetry of language dominance, when processing language they will have less of an innate tendency to scan in the correct left to right direction (Heilman, 1980).

Orton proposed a dominance hypothesis in which visual images in each hemisphere are mirror images of each other. He thought that in normal people, the images lying in the nondominant hemisphere became suppressed (not seen). In dyslexic children, dominance is less strong and the minor hemisphere is not suppressed, which induces both mirror writing and reading (Simner, 1984).

One of the theories of kinetic reversals of young children is The Grammar of Action Theory. According to this theory, there appears to be a uniformity in stroke sequence and direction that kindergarten children use when they copy geometric figures. This stems from an underlying system of strongly ingrained motor rules that is referred to as a *grammar of action*. Certain left-right mirror image reversals errors that occur from time to time when children print letters and numbers might result from an occasional misapplication of these motor rules. It is proposed that the letters that require children to amend their normal use of these motor rules when they print should be reversed more frequently than letters that can be formed in a manner that is compatible with the child's motor rule

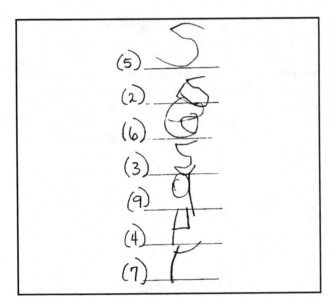

Figure 9-1. Reversals.

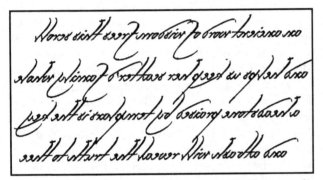

Figure 9-3. Mirror writing. From Brown, D. *The DaVinci code.* New York: Doubleday. Reprinted with permission.

Figure 9-2. An N can be reversed to the figure shown.

letters or words backward and not others. These are not errors of orientation or direction but are more accurately classified as errors in letter sequence. It has been stated that among second and third grade poor readers, reversals of letter orientation such as b/d and reversals of letter order such as was/saw were not covariant but constitutes two distinct categories of reading errors (Moyer, 1977).

The reversing of letters due to stroke sequence is a totally different reversal error and represents a third category. Mirror writing may accompany neurological disease but it is also produced by normal individuals. Mirror writing is seen in various disorders affecting the central nervous system, for example, Parkinson's disease. Acquired mirror writing most commonly follows cerebrovascular lesions in the left hemisphere. Almost all mirror writing is done with the left hand. Many normal mirror writers are or were originally left-handed.

There have been several famous people who were mirror writers. Leonardo da Vinci is notably the most celebrated mirror writer (Figure 9-3). He was left-handed and his cerebral dominance for writing might have been in the right hemisphere. He also wrote some letters in normal script. The direction in which Leonardo's normal script was written and whether he used his right or left hand will never be known. Almost all of Leonard's huge literary output was written from right to left in mirror script, although numerals appear in both mirror and normal form (McMonnies, 1992). Lewis Carroll, author of *Alice in Wonderland* and *Through the Looking Glass*, was also known to write at times in mirror writing (Schott, 1999).

I am concluding this chapter with a basic type of reversal remediation. You should become familiar with its format and why different stages are used. Don't go on to the next stage until the one you are on is mastered. It is important that you are familiar with this section before going on with a remediation program.

Basic Type of Reversal Remediation

Stage I (The Discrimination Stage)

Have the child become familiar with the four main transformations that confuse young children. He is to match the sample at the left to one of the four examples.

system. For right-handed children, the printing demands associated with d but not b contradict the rule that states that all horizontal lines should start at the left and be drawn towards the right (Simner, 1984). Therefore, d is reversed more than b. The Grammar of Action rules are as follows for a right-handed child.

1. Start at a left most point.
2. Start at a topmost point.
3. Given a figure with an apex, start at the top and come down the left oblique. This rule applies to only these designs (triangle, diamond, inverted V).
4. Draw all horizontal lines from left to right.
5. Draw all vertical lines from top to bottom.
6. Thread, i. e., draw with a continuous line. Don't take the pencil off of the page. This is why an N can be reversed to the figure shown in Figure 9-2. (Goodnow, 1973; Simner, 1984).

Word pair reversals such as on/no, saw/was do not form mirror images. It is unlikely that a child would see some

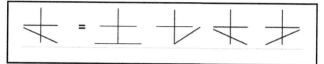

Figure 9-4. Line tilt.

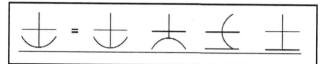

Figure 9-5. Line to curve.

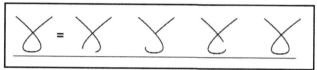

Figure 9-6. Break and close.

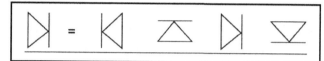

Figure 9-7. Rotation and close.

    a. Line tilt (Match Figure 9-4)
    b. Line to curve (Match Figure 9-5)
    c. Break and close (Match Figure 9-6)
    d. Rotation and close (Match Figure 9-7)

Once you feel the child understands and can do these exercises, proceed to Stage 2.

Stage 2 (Matching to Sample Task)

This is a simultaneous matching to sample task. The child should select from among b, d, p and of the letter that matches in the orientation to a sample letter; for example, b. Match sample b with d p d b p.

Stage 3 (Matching From Memory)

Same as Stage 2, but the child must remember the sample and then find its match. For example, match b with d p d b p. He looks at the sample for 5 seconds and then finds its match from memory. Use the same sample letter for several trials.

Stage 4 (Letter Names)

When matching from direction of the letters is automatic, the child should be taught the letter names. Don't confuse him at the beginning with too much memory work. For example, show the child a "b". Have him name it and then find it in a sequence of letters (d p d b p q).

Stage 5 (Train in Pairs)

For example, point to the side the circle is on: bb bd db bd. When this is mastered, have him also name the letter after he points to the correct side.

Stage 6 (Train in Context)

Have the child find as many words as he can out of a magazine that has a b or d and have him name the letter.

Stage 7 (Color Coding)

Have the child color in red all the b's and color in blue all the d's from a page in a magazine. Do the same with p and q.

Stage 8 (Scanning Patterns)

Where a child starts his visual scan is important. Draw large letters on the board and number in sequence the proper scanning patterns of top to bottom and left to right. At the beat of a metronome, the child calls out the numbers in proper sequence and ends it by saying the name of the letter or numbers. For an example, see Figure 9-8.

Stage 9

Transposing letters within a word and adding or substituting letters.

    1. Vowel-consonant reversals are more common on short words, while omissions are more common on long words.
    2. Vowel and consonant errors far exceed the incidence of reversals of sequence and orientation.

These errors are probably due to poor reading skills. They are not mirror images. The principle source of reading errors that cause reversals in words of dyslexic children is probably due to difficulties in phonetic segmentation of words in the lexicon (storing), in phonic recoding (retrieving), and in mastery of orthography (spelling patterns). In short, these children have linguistic problems, not perceptual problems. Children who substitute letters or reverse a couple of letters need a strong phonics program. Teach the child phonics rules.

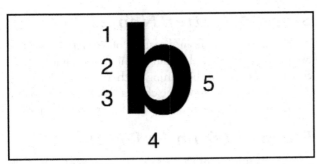

Figure 9-8. Scanning patterns.

Stage 10 (Word Reversals)

Reversing the entire word is due to poor reading and scanning skills because the child is reading one word at a time and scanning right to left. The child needs to be taught left to right scanning and to be trained in context. For example, "I stopped by the store on my way home". If the child was reading this sentence properly, he would not switch *no* for *on*. He must be taught the overall meaning of the sentence or paragraph. For example, we all went to the zoo after lunch. I saw a monkey. The child who has good understanding of these sentences would not switch *was* for *saw*. Show the child commonly reversed words like *was* and *on*. Have him practice left to right scanning by calling the letters out in sequence. Also, use other words and have him call the letters out in left to right sequence.

References

Fischer, W. F. (1971). *Reading reversals and developmental dyslexia: A further study.* Storrs, CT: University of Connecticut; 486-510.

Frith, U. (1971). Why do children reverse letters? *British Journal of Psychology, 62,* 459-468.

Goodnow, J. J. (1973). The grammar of action: Sequence and syntax in children's copying. *Cognitive Psychology,* 82-98.

Harman, S. (1982). Are reversals a symptom of dyslexia? *The Reading Teacher,* 424-428.

Heilman, K. M. (1980). Mirror-reading and writing in association with right-left spatial disorientation. *Journal of Neurology, Neurosurgery and Psychiatry, 143,* 774-780.

Kaufman, N. L. (1980). Review of research on reversal errors. *Perceptual and Motor Skills, 51,* 55-79.

McMonnies, C. W. (1992). Visuo-spatial discrimination and mirror image letter reversals in reading. *Journal of the American Optometric Association,* 698-704.

Moyer, S. B. (1977). Reversals in reading: Diagnosis and remediation. *Exceptional Children,* 424-429.

Schott, G. D. (1999). Mirror writing: Allen's self observations. Lewis Carroll's "looking glass" letters and Leonardo Da Vinci's maps. Journal: Department of history. *The Lance, V354,* 2158-2161.

Simner, M. L. (1984). The grammar of action and reversal errors in children's printing. *Developmental Psychology, 20,* 136-142.

Wallace, J. R. (2001). Spatial perspective. Taking errors in children. *Perceptual and Motor Skills, 92,* 633-639.

Form Rev-1
LETTER ORIENTATION

Purpose: Reversals.

Materials: Marker board, magazine pictures.

Method: Have the child do the following activities.

Level 1: Cut pictures from a magazine and turn them in different directions. Ask the child if they are backwards or not. Ask him if it makes a difference for the identification of the picture if it is backwards or not. Show him the orientation of letters and explain how their orientation is important for identification but not pictures.

Level 2: Draw letters or numbers on the blackboard. Have some facing in the wrong direction. Have him circle the ones that are wrong and have him draw them the proper way.

Level 3: Have the child circle certain letters in a line of print from a magazine. For example, all the b's or d's.

Level 4: Draw some letters on the board. Ask him to draw the letter as it would look if it was turned halfway to the right or left, upside down, etc.

Form Rev-2
B-D-P-Q Sorting

Purpose: Reversals.

Materials: b-d-p-q Sorting Chart, metronome, balance disc or walking rail.

Method: Place the b-d-p-q Sorting Chart at eye level on the wall.

Level 2: The child stands in front of the chart and touches each letter as he calls it out, going from left to right or top to bottom.

Level 3:
1. Child stands in front of the chart and names each letter to the beat of the metronome.
2. Have the child touch and name any one letter. For example, all b's or all d's to the beat of the metronome.
3. Do #2 with right hand and then with left hand.
4. Alternate hands. Touch the first letter with his right hand and call it out, then touch the second letter with his left hand and call it out.

Level 4:
1. Child stands on balance disc or end of walking rail in front of chart. He is to call out the sounds the letters make instead of the names of the letters. For example, the "buh" sound or "duh" sound or "puh" sound.
2. Call out the names of every other letter or every third letter. Do in both vertical and horizontal directions.
3. Go left to right and call out the name of the letter and say the direction the loop is facing. For example, q left, b right.

b-d-p-q Sorting Chart

q	b	p	d	b	p	q
d	p	d	q	p	d	p
p	d	p	b	d	b	d
d	p	q	d	b	d	p
b	d	p	q	d	p	b
p	b	d	p	b	p	d
b	p	b	d	p	q	p
p	d	q	p	b	d	b
q	b	d	b	d	q	d

Form Rev-3
DIRECTIONAL "U" SACCADES

Purpose: Reversals.

Materials: Directional "U" worksheet.

Method: Set the metronome at 60 beats per minute (slower or faster if desired). The child stands 20 feet away from the worksheet, which is hung on the wall.

Level 1: Tell the child to clasp his hands together and extend them in front of himself. To each beat of the metronome, he is to move his hands in the direction of the opening in each U. Do each line in a left to right manner.

Level 2:
1. Tell the child to clasp his hands together and extend them in front of himself. To each beat of the metronome, he is to move his hands in the direction of the opening in each U and call out the directions (right, left, up or down). Do each line in a left to right manner.
2. Repeat #1, going down the vertical columns from top to bottom.
3. Without the metronome and without using his hands, see how fast he can do both the horizontal and vertical rows and call out the direction of each opening.

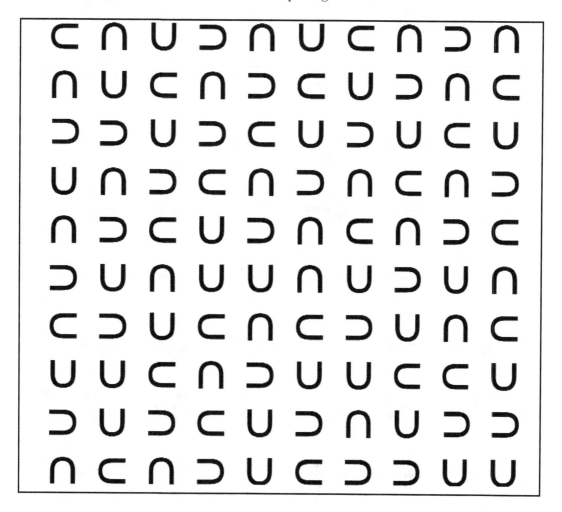

Form Rev-4
Directional Arrows

Purpose: Reversals.

Materials: Metronome, Directional Arrows worksheet.

Method: The child is seated at a table next to you. Have him hold the worksheet at normal reading distance.

Level 1:
1. At the beat of the metronome, the child is to name the direction of each arrow. Start on the horizontal line and move in a left to right sequence.
2. Same as #1, but go down the vertical lines from top to bottom.
3. Without the metronome, time him and see how fast he can do the horizontal and vertical lines.

Level 2: At the beat of the metronome, the child is to walk in a heel to toe manner on the walking rail. As he walks, have him call out the direction of the arrows. Go in both the horizontal direction and the vertical direction.

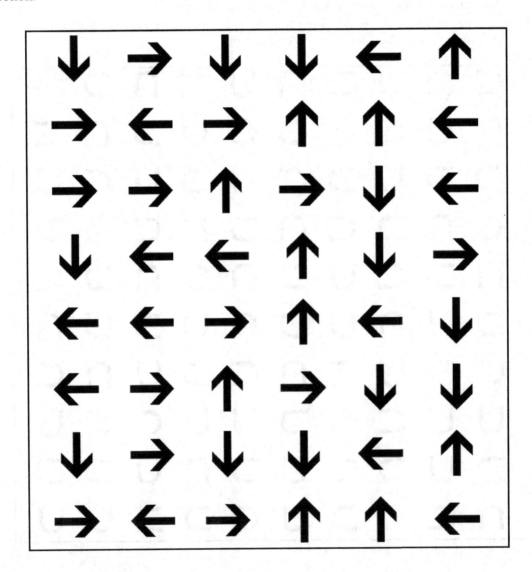

Form Rev-5
TEACH LETTERS BY CLASSES

Purpose: Reversals.

Materials: Marker board.

Method: On the marker board, show the child all the letters in the alphabet by classes. For example, all the letters with loops to the right, loops to the left, letters with horizontal lines, vertical lines, lines that cross and curved lines.

Level 1: Have the child practice drawing all the letters of the alphabet on the marker board by classes.

Level 2: Tell the child which class of letters you want him to find and have him circle them in a book or magazine.

Form Rev-6
FLASH CARDS AND REVERSED LETTERS

Purpose: Reversals.

Materials: 3 inch x 5 inch index cards.

Method: Print in lower case letters, words from the child's Instant Words List on index cards. Print one word per card. Purposely reverse letters in about half of the words. Have the remaining words correct with no letters reversed.

Level 2:
1. Give the child the flash cards one at a time. He is to study the card and tell you whether the card has an error or not. If it does contain an error, he circles it and then writes the word correctly on a marker board or piece of paper.
2. Flash each card to the child for about 3 seconds. Have him tell you if any of the letters were reversed or not. Have him correctly print any word that had a letter reversed in it.

Instant Words List

These are the words most used in reading and writing English, grouped in order of frequency of use.

1	2	3	4	5	6
the	he	go	who	saw	big
a	I	see	an	home	where
is	they	then	their	soon	am
you	one	us	she	stand	ball
to	good	no	new	box	morning
and	me	him	said	upon	live
we	about	by	did	first	four
that	had	was	boy	came	last
in	if	come	three	girl	color
not	some	get	down	house	away
for	up	or	work	find	red
at	her	two	put	because	friend
with	do	man	were	made	pretty
it	when	little	before	could	eat
on	so	has	just	book	want
can	my	them	long	look	year
will	very	how	here	mother	white
are	all	like	other	run	got
of	would	our	old	school	play
this	any	what	take	people	found
your	been	know	cat	night	left
as	out	make	again	into	men
but	there	which	give	say	bring
be	from	much	after	think	wish
have	day	his	many	back	black

Form Rev-6 (continued)
FLASH CARDS AND REVERSED LETTERS

7	8	9	10	11	12
may	ran	ask	hat	off	fire
let	five	small	car	sister	ten
use	read	yellow	write	happy	order
these	over	show	try	once	part
right	such	goes	myself	didn't	early
present	way	clean	longer	set	fat
tell	too	buy	those	round	third
next	shall	thank	hold	dress	same
please	own	sleep	full	fall	love
leave	most	letter	carry	wash	hear
hand	sure	jump	eight	start	yesterday
more	thing	help	sing	always	eyes
why	only	fly	warm	anything	door
better	near	don't	sit	around	clothes
under	than	fast	dog	close	though
while	open	cold	ride	walk	o'clock
should	kind	today	hot	money	second
never	must	does	grow	turn	water
each	high	face	cut	might	town
best	far	green	seven	hard	took
another	both	every	woman	along	pair
seem	end	brown	funny	bed	now
tree	also	coat	yes	fine	keep
name	until	six	ate	sat	head
dear	call	gave	stop	hope	food

Form Rev-7
FILL IN THE LOOPS

Purpose: Reversals.

Materials: Book or magazine, red pen, blue pen.

Method: Have the child do the following activities.

Level 3:
1. Use a page from a book or magazine. The child is to fill in all the loops of letters facing the right with red and all the loops of letters facing left with blue.
2. Time him. See how quickly he can complete a page without missing any loops.

Level 4:
1. Use a page from a book or magazine. The child is to fill in all the loops of letters facing the right in red and facing left in blue.
2. Once the child can do #1, instead of filling in the loops, he is to call out the letter and which color he would have used to fill in the loop.

Form Rev-8
THE BED

Purpose: Reversals.

Materials: None.

Method: Explain to the child that the loop on the "b" faces to the right. Hold his left hand in front of him with his thumb pointing to the right. For example:

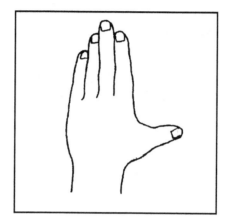

Explain how the loop on the "d" faces to the left. Hold his left hand in front of him with his thumb pointing to the left. For example:

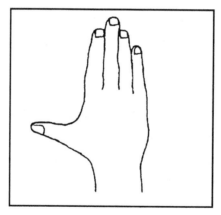

Form Rev-8 (continued)
THE BED

Level 2: A good way for the child to remember the direction of the b and d is to have him hold his two hands together to from a bed. Have him practice spelling "bed". For example:

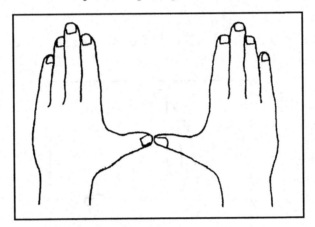

The left hand with the thumb pointing to the right is the "b", the right hand with the thumb pointing to the left is the "d".

Form Rev-9
VECTORS

Purpose: Reversals.

Materials: Marker board, protractor.

Method: A vector is a straight line drawn at different angles. For example:

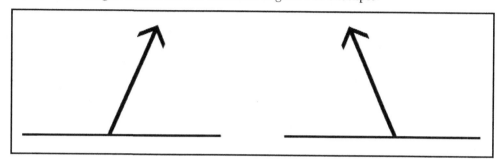

On the board, draw several vectors. Show the child how the angle can change between the vector and the straight horizontal line.

Level 2: On the blackboard, draw a vector. Have the child draw one like yours next to it on the board. It must be close to the same angle as the one you have drawn. Draw several in different positions for the child to copy.

Level 3:

1. Make letters on the board. Show the child how vectors can be part of a letter. For example:

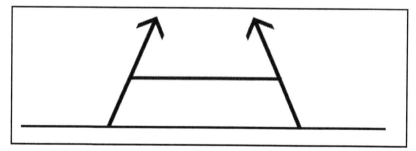

2. Draw a vector. Have the child make a letter out of it. For example:

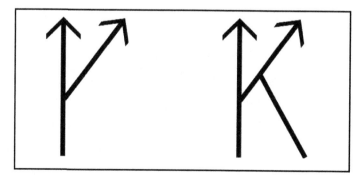

Form Rev-9 (continued)
VECTORS

Level 4:
1. Make a vector on a piece of paper. Have the child make one just like it with his protractor.
2. Draw a vector on the paper with the protractor. The child must make a vector with the same angle but in the opposite direction.

Form Rev-10
COMMONLY REVERSED WORDS

Purpose: Reversals.

Materials: 3 inch x 5 inch index cards, marker board.

Method: The following are commonly reversed words: on, no, saw, was, not, ton, dam, mad, rat, tar, pot, top, bat, tab, wed, dew, mug, gum, pit, tip.

Level 4A:
1. Have the child make cards with commonly reversed words. Then have the child finger trace the word while saying it. Next, remove the card and have the child write the word from memory. Repeat this procedure until the child can read and write the word several times without error.
2. Use one of the words in a sentence and have the child indicate the same word on the card.

Level 4B:
1. Make a list of commonly reversed words with one word over the paired reversed word, allowing some space between the two pairs. Then have him draw a line between similar letters. For example:

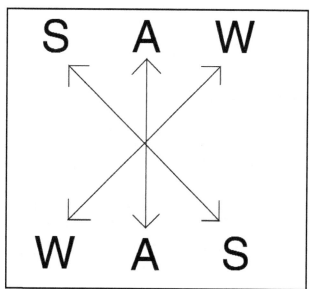

2. On an index card, print or write one of the commonly reversed words. Purposely miswrite a letter in some of the words. For example, "toq" instead of "top". The child is to tell you whether the word looks right or wrong and why.

Form Rev-11
DISTINCTIVE FEATURES

Purpose: Reversals.

Materials: Marker board, magazine pictures, metronome, plastic or wooden letters.

Method: Have the child do the following activities.

Level 1:
1. Show the child a picture from a magazine. Ask him questions about the picture. For example, how many cars are in the picture? What color are they? What is the man in the picture wearing?
2. Show the child two different pictures of the same object. For example, cars. Ask him how the two pictures are different.

Level 2A:
Draw letters on the marker board. Make them large and put numbers next to the letter so that as the child looks at the numbers in sequence, he will be scanning the letter in the proper top to bottom or left to right direction. For example:

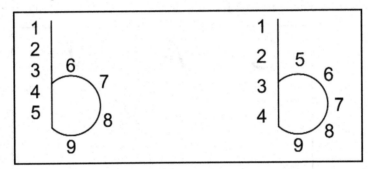

At each beat of the metronome, have him move his eyes to the next number. Train all capital and lower case letters together.

Level 2B:
Have the child group the alphabet by classes. For example, all letters with loops, with curves, with diagonal lines, with just vertical and horizontal lines. Make sure he knows what vertical, horizontal, and diagonal mean. Have him draw the letters on the marker board.

Level 3A:
1. Draw part of a letter on the board. Have the child tell you what letter it is. When you do this, use mainly horizontal and vertical lines as these are the lines that give us the most information for letter recognition.
2. In a line of letters from a book, have him circle all the letters with vertical, horizontal, or diagonal lines.
3. Show the child a picture from a magazine. Have him find as many angles, curves, horizontal, vertical, and diagonal lines as possible. Ask him what letters these could make.

Level 3B:
1. Have the child describe how one letter is different from another.
2. When a child draws a letter, have him verbally describe it. for example, as he draws a "b", he describes the vertical line and the loop that is attached to the lower right side.

Form Rev-11 (continued)
DISTINCTIVE FEATURES

Level 3C:
1. Letter counting: on a line of letters from a book, have the child count how many of certain letters there are. For example, how many b's or d's, etc.
2. With his eyes closed, have the child feel upper and lower case plastic or wooden letters and tell you which letter he is feeling. Have him describe the letter.

Level 4A: Write some letters on the marker board. Ask him which letter does not belong in the group. For example, N, W, K, P. The answer would be a P because it is the only letter with a loop.

Level 4B:
1. Have the child find as many different styles of print as he can. Ask him how the letters are different for each style. Ask him how they are the same.
2. Have the child look at the page of a book. Have him describe how certain words are shaped alike. For example, same length, start with the same letter, have a lot of letters with loops, etc.

Level 5: Ask him how many ways he can describe the parts of a letter. For example, b could be described: vertical line, curved line, closed loop at the bottom of the letter, vertical line to the left of the loop. The letter N could be described: two vertical lines, one vertical line to the left of the diagonal, one vertical line to the right of the diagonal, two small angles where the lines intersect, the diagonal line touches the top of the left vertical line and the bottom of the right vertical line.

Form Rev-12
BILATERAL CIRCLES

Purpose: Reversals.

Materials: Marker board, metronome.

Method: An X is placed at nose height in front of the child on a marker board. The child stands and looks at the X while being visually and physically aware of what his arms and hands are doing as he moves his arms to draw large circles on the marker board. The circles should be about 12 inches in diameter.

Level 1: Have the child stand in front of the marker board and look at the X. The X should be at nose level directly in front of him. Have the child practice drawing circles one level at a time. He should try to make the circles as round as possible and stay on the same line. Have him do it first with his right hand and then his left.

Level 2:
1. The child's first task is to figure out the four different combinations of directions the arms can move while making two circles simultaneously. He is helped as little as possible in figuring this out. The goal is to have him be able to work out the logic that the hands can go different ways—two ways in the same direction and two ways in the opposite direction. For example:

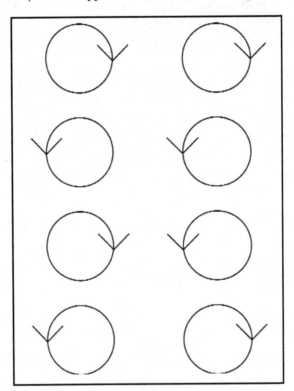

2. Practice having him draw the two circles at the same time. Practice having him move his arms in the four different directions. Try to have him make the circles as close to the same size as possible.

Form Rev-12 (continued)
BILATERAL CIRCLES

Level 3:

1. Draw a vertical line at the top and at the bottom of each circle.

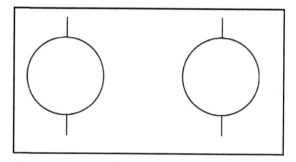

As he draws around the circles and the marker comes to the top line, he is to say "top" and when it comes to the bottom line, he is to say "bottom".

2. The metronome is added. On the first beat, he should have the marker at the top line and say "top", on the second beat, he should have moved the marker at a speed that will have it at the bottom line and he says "bottom".

3. Same activities as #1 and 2, but one circle may be higher, lower, larger, or smaller than the other.

Level 4: Two circles are placed on the board in front of the child. Two lines are placed vertically and horizontally. Use the metronome. For example:

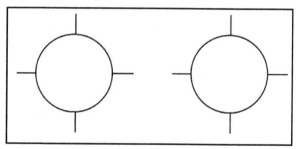

The child makes circles in each of the four different directions his arms can move. (Two in the same direction and two in the opposite direction.) As he comes to each line, at the beat of the metronome he says the position of the chalk so that in addition to "top" and "bottom", he says "right" and "left" when both hands are on the sides of the circles. When the hands are going in the opposite direction, he says "in" and "out" instead of "right" and "left".

Form Rev-12 (continued)
BILATERAL CIRCLES

Level 5: The procedure involves one circle with four lines dividing it into quarters and one with three lines dividing it into thirds. The circles are about 12 inches in diameter. For example:

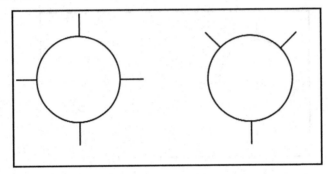

The child's hands go around the circles in the four different directions; two in the same direction and two in the opposite direction. Each hand is to reach the next line on the next beat of the metronome. One hand must travel faster than the other to attain accuracy. No words are to be said as he completes this procedure. One hand traces the circle in four beats while the other is doing it in three beats. These circles can also be made in different sizes as well as different heights on the board.

Form Rev-13
MARKER BOARD SQUARES

Purpose: Reversals.

Materials: Marker board, metronome.

Method: An X is placed at nose height on the board in front of the child. Two squares about 12 inches in size are placed on either side of the X. For example:

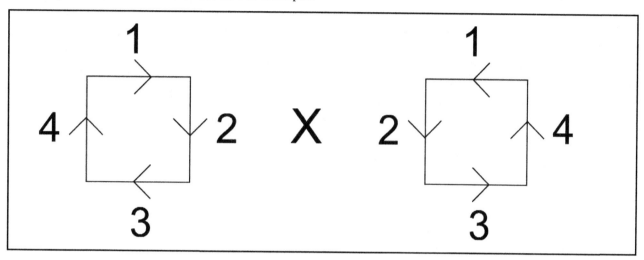

Level 1: Have the child stand in front of the X with the X at nose level. Have him practice tracing the squares. Have him trace the right square with his right hand and the left square with his left. He is to try and stay on the lines.

Level 2:
1. Have the child start in the same corner of each square. Make both hands follow the lines to each corner of the squares, first in one direction and then in the opposite direction.
2. Have him do #1, but call out the direction in which his hands are going.

Level 3:
1. Have the left hand start at the top left corner of the left square, and the right hand at the top right corner of the right square. The instructions are: "make your hands go in two different directions, calling out the directions the hands are going as you move them". The right hand will go from right to left and the left hand from left to right. The child would say "in, down, out and up". The next direction would be both hands going "down" and then in toward each other saying, "in, up, out". This gives four different directions for tracing squares.
2. Same as #1, but a metronome is set at 40 beats. The child is told to be at a corner each time the metronome beats, and say the direction that the hands move.

Level 4:
1. Have the child put both hands at the top left corner of each square and go in opposite directions. This is done at the beat of the metronome (40 beats a minute), but without saying the direction in which the hands are going. For instance, starting at the top left of both squares, the right hand goes right and the left down. On the next beat, the right hand goes down and the left goes right.
2. Same as #1, but make squares of different sizes and heights on the board.

Form Rev-14
FIGURE EIGHTS

Purpose: Reversals.

Materials: Marker board, metronome.

Method: Two eights at 12 inches apart and about 2 feet tall are placed at each side of an X drawn at nose height. On the marker board, a vertical line is drawn at the top and bottom of both eights and a horizontal line through the middle of the eights. For example:

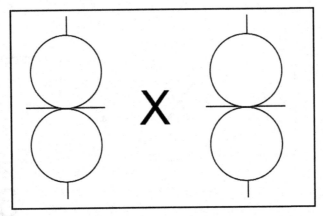

Level 1: Have the child stand in front of the X when it is at nose level. He is to trace the right figure eight with his right hand and the left with his left hand. He is to try and stay on the lines.

Level 2:
1. The child stands and looks at the X. He is to figure out the four different combinations of directions the arms can move while tracing the two eights simultaneously. For example:

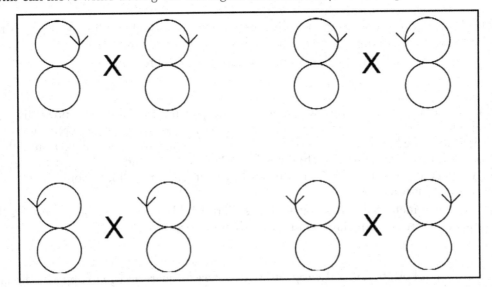

2. Same as #1, but use the metronome and have the child call out the directions his hands are moving. For example: "top", "middle" and "bottom" as he crosses the lines on each beat of the metronome.
3. Make the eights different sizes and do the same as #2.

Form Rev-14 (continued)
FIGURE EIGHTS

Level 3:

1. Draw the eights on their sides (lazy eights). For example:

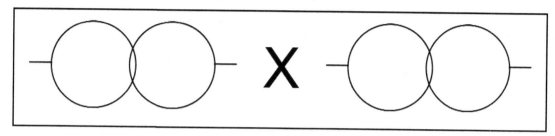

A metronome is used while the child calls out the direction his hands move. For example, if both hands start at the left line and move up, he will call out "top", "middle", "bottom", "side".

2. Set the metronome at a slow beat. At each beat he is to be at the horizontal lines. He doesn't have to call out directions.

3. Vary the locations the hands start from. For example, one hand can start on the left side of the left figure eight and the other hand can start on the right side of the right figure eight. Use the metronome at a slow rate.

Form Rev-15
TRIANGLE AND SQUARE

Purpose: Reversals.

Materials: Marker board, metronome.

Method: Put an X on the board at nose height in front of the child. Draw a square and a triangle on either side of the X. The square and triangle are about 1 foot in height. For example:

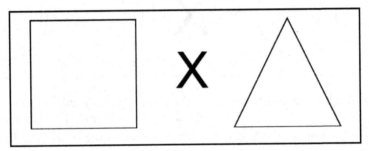

Level 3: Have the child trace the lines of each figure simultaneously. The metronome is used but the child is not to name the direction of the hands, because one hand makes three different directional movements to complete the task and the other makes four. Have the child figure out the four different directions that the two figures can be traced.

Form Rev-16
FELT LETTERS

Purpose: To eliminate letter or number reversals.

Materials: A "felt" board—a square board covered in felt. The board should be about 2 feet by 2 feet. Numerous letters and numbers made one side only out of felt. When you see a number or letter the child often reverses, cover the side that goes on the board with something other than felt. For example, if he often reverses or confuses the number 7, put a smooth surface over the felt on the side that goes on the board.

Method: Have the child do math exercises using the felt board and felt numbers. For example:

$$\begin{array}{r} 16 \\ +17 \\ \hline 33 \end{array}$$

If he puts the 7 on the board in the wrong direction, it will fall off.

Form Rev-17
MAGAZINE LETTER HUNT

Purpose: To help eliminate reversals.

Materials: Old magazines.

Method: Have the child look at a magazine that is lying on a table in front of him. He is to start at the top row at the far left position. Have him (while scanning left to right) find and circle as many words as he can that have a b or d or p or q in the first position. After he circles them, he starts a flashcard list of all the words he has circled. That will be his sight word list. (You decide which words will be added to his sight word list, as some may be too difficult for him.)

Level 2: Have the child circle the words. Do not do a word list.

Levels 3 to 5: Do the activity described in the Method section above.

Chapter Ten

EXAMPLES OF DAILY LESSON PLANS

I am including four lesson plans that you can use as an example on how to design your own lessons. You will give your child five activities each day that he will work on for 10 minutes each. From the questionnaire that the parents complete (see Appendix) and a good case history, you will decide on which areas need the most attention. I suggest that you include at least one motor and one ocular motor exercise each day.

The questionnaire will help you get started on designing your daily lesson plans. Pick the areas that are in the questions that have been answered with "always". The first problem area after the question that is underlined is the main area for that question. The other ones are subordinate areas. Do three activities a day from the main area of concern and two from the subordinate areas. If no question is answered as "always", use "frequently".

I have given you only 1 month of activities as an example. The average child will probably be in therapy from nine months to 1 year. You must keep the child interested by varying the activities while continuing to work on the main problem areas.

The key to success is a good case history and your knowledge of the problem areas. Each chapter in my book was designed to give you technical knowledge to help you understand why you are using these activities.

Example 1

During the course of your case history, the parents of this 7-year-old first grade male tell you the following:
1. Slight delay in motor but not bad—perhaps a few months
2. Just learned to ride his two wheeler without training wheels
3. Tends to avoid sports activities
4. Tells you he doesn't like sports
5. Now starting to have difficulty in school, especially in areas that require sequencing such as phonics.

This case history should alert you that this child probably has gross motor difficulties. As in any lesson plan, spend about two-thirds of the time on the major area and the other third on subordinate areas. In this case, the subordinate areas would be ocular motor and visual motor perception. Start at Level 2.

Lesson Plan 1

12 sessions at 3 times per week for 1 month:

Day 1	Day 2	Day 3	Day 4
GM 20	GM 20	GM 5	GM 8
GM 21	GM 21	GM 7	GM 16
GM 10	GM 10	GM 18	GM 18
VM 6	OM 13	OM 21	VMP 8
VMP 18	OM 20	OM 6	VMP 6

Day 5	Day 6	Day 7	Day 8
GM 23	GM 20	GM 22	GM 29
GM 6	GM 18	GM 23	GM 18
GM 20	GM 22	GM 25	GM 9
VMP 28	OM 14	OM 21	VMP 6
OM 17	OM 16	OM 8	OM 20

Day 9	Day 10	Day 11	Day 12
GM 9	GM 25	GM 16	GM 22
GM 18	GM 22	GM 13	GM 25
GM 17	GM 16	GM 20	GM 5
VMP 6	VMP 7	VMP 16	OM 24
OM 20	OM 20	OM 21	OM 17

Example 2

This child is 8 years old and is in second grade. His mother reports that he's always had difficulty copying from the board and is often the last child finished copying his assignments. He also uses his finger for a marker and reports letters and words moving as he reads. As you might expect, he is a very slow reader.

This child's main problem is ocular motor skills. There are probably some gross motor and visual motor perception problems as well. Start at Level 2.

Lesson Plan 2

Day 1	Day 2	Day 3	Day 4
OM 6	OM 20	OM 6	OM 20
OM 20	OM 21	OM 12	OM 12
OM 8	OM 6	OM 8	OM 22
GM 4	GM 4	GM 13	GM 13
GM 22	GM 22	GM 29	GM 29

Day 5	Day 6	Day 7	Day 8
OM 20	OM 21	OM 21	OM 16
OM 21	OM 16	OM 16	OM 21
OM 22	OM 17	OM 17	OM 25
GM 16	GM 16	GM 18	GM 18
GM 20	GM 20	GM 20	VMP 7

Day 9	Day 10	Day 11	Day 12
OM 16	OM 22	OM 22	OM 22
OM 21	OM 10	OM 21	OM 10
OM 25	OM 21	OM 25	OM 21
GM 22	GM 22	GM 21	GM 21
VMP 8	GM 25	GM 29	GM 20

Lesson Plan 3

This 7-year-old first grade student has been sent to you because of reversals. According to her mother, all children reverse at times, but Wendy is excessive, she still reverses individual numbers and letters. Her school grades are only fair, and her mother feels they would be much better if she didn't reverse as much as she does. Obviously, our main area here is reversals, but add laterality and visual memory to it. Start at Level 1.

For the first 6 days, follow the lesson plan at the end of the chapter on Reversals. We will call this GP or General Plan.

Day 1	Day 2	Day 3	Day 4
REV (GP)	REV (GP)	REV (GP)	REV (GP)
REV (GP)	REV (GP)	REV (GP)	REV (GP)
REV (GP)	REV (GP)	REV (GP)	REV (GP)
L 7	L 6	L 10	L 7
VM 2	VM 9	VM 7	VM 12

Day 5	Day 6	Day 7	Day 8
REV (GP)	REV (GP)	REV (GP)	REV (GP)
REV (GP)	REV (GP)	REV (GP)	REV (GP)
REV (GP)	REV (GP)	REV (GP)	REV (GP)
L 7	L 19	L 10	L 11
VM 16	L 11	L 11	L 12

Day 9	Day 10	Day 11	Day 12
REV 14	REV 17	REV 16	REV 16
REV 5	REV 2	REV 2	REV 4
REV 4	REV 3	REV 3	REV 3
L 19	L 19	VM 23	VM 20
VM 25	VM 23	L 8	L 15

Lesson Plan 4

We will call this our general lesson plan. In this plan, we have a 6-year-old boy who can't seem to do anything correctly. He has poor motor, very poor ocular motor and visual motor perception. He still reverses and has very poor visual memory skills. I will list some of my favorite activities in this lesson plan. A general plan like this one should have a motor and ocular motor activity in each day's plan. Start at Level 1.

Day 1	Day 2	Day 3	Day 4
GM 20	GM 20	GM 20	GM 21
OM 20	OM 20	OM 21	OM 21
VM 1	VM 4	VM 5	VM 7
L 20	L 20	L 19	L 19
VMP 6	REV 2	VMP 9	REV 7

Day 5	Day 6	Day 7	Day 8
GM 22	GM 25	GM 21	GM 18
OM 22	OM 22	OM 22	OM 8
VM 7	VM 15	VM 17	VM 16
L 10	L 10	L 15	L 15
VMP 10	REV 11	VMP 13	REV 16

Day 9	Day 10	Day 11	Day 12
GM 18	GM 22	GM 22	GM 20
OM 8	OM 21	OM 20	OM 21
VM 26	VM 26	VM 25	VM 6
L 6	L 4	L 7	L 7
REV 16	VMP 33	VMP 14	REV 2

Glossary of Terms

allele: One or two alternative forms of a gene, occupying corresponding sites.

balance board: A square or round board about two and one-half feet in diameter. The board is balanced on a piece of wood about six inches in diameter and tapered to about three inches. The child stands on the board to improve his balance skills.

brainstem: The stemlike portion of the brain connecting the cerebral hemispheres with the spinal cord.

cerebellum: A part of the brain that occupies the posterior cranial fossa behind the brain stem. It is concerned with the coordination of movements, especially eye-hand coordination and eye movements.

cerebral cortex: The thin layer of gray matter on the surface of the cerebral hemisphere. It is responsible for our higher mental functions including reading and perception.

cognitive processing: Includes all aspects of perceiving, thinking and remembering.

context clues: Help us understand what we are reading as a result of being familiar with the topic or theme we are reading about.

corporal potentiality: Excluding bodily interference in order to obtain higher learning processes.

cortical: Same as cerebral cortex.

dextral: Right.

directionality: Understanding an external object's proper orientation (i.e., the proper orientation of letters and numbers).

feature detectors: Are located in the fovea and are probably the cones. They are used to discriminate the different features of letters for letter and word identification.

fine motor: Refers to activities that require small muscle movements (i.e., eye movements, writing, etc.).

fixation: The act of directing the eyes to the object we are looking at so that the image of the object can be centered on the fovea.

fixation chart: A chart with rows of numbers on it.

fixation point: The object of which the eyes are directed to during a fixation, (i.e., a letter in a word).

fovea: The small 1.5 mm area of the retina where the cones are located. This is the area of the retina where we get our color vision and sharp visual acuity. Light must focus on this area for clear vision.

grapheme: A minimal unit of a writing system.

gross motor: Refers to the activities that require large muscle movements (i.e., walking, balancing, hopping, etc.).

homozygotes: Possessing a pair of identical alleles at a given locus.

laterality: The internal awareness of the two sides of the body and their differences. For a child, this is his ability to know his right side from his left.

letter chart: A chart with rows of letters on it.

Marsden ball: A ball, 2 to 3 inches in diameter, hung from the ceiling by a string. It is used in many motor and vision training procedures.

metronome: An instrument for beating a desired time. It is used as an aid in practicing music.

motor skills: Includes both gross and fine motor skills.

ocular motor: Pertains to movements of the eyes, especially movements involved in following a moving object or scanning words in a "left" to "right" direction while reading.

orthography: Spelling patterns. The art of understanding the proper positions of letters in words.

perception: Recognition and identification of our environment. Visual perception would be visual recognition and identification of our environment.

perceptual motor: Refers to perceptual and motor skills. Perceptual development is accomplished through motor involvement.

peripheral vision: Refers to vision other than central vision. As we look at an object, the area to the side of what we are looking at is in our peripheral vision.

phoneme: Any of the minimal units of speech sound in a language that can serve to distinguish one word from another.

regression: Indicates rereading. Any time the eye moves back to the left, instead of the right, as we read across a page.

saccadic eye movements: Rapid, accurate eye movement from fixation point to fixation point.

semantics: Knowledge of word meaning.

sequential processing: The ability to process information given to you a little at time in consecutive order. Children who have problems in sequential processing have difficulty remembering things in sequence (i.e., the letters in the alphabet or lists of spelling words).

simultaneous processing: The ability to process many pieces of information given to you all at once. Children who have simultaneous processing problems may have poor reading comprehension skills.

span of recognition: The amount of print that the brain can recognize during a single fixation.

sustained activity: The neurological activity that processes the visual information of the letters and words we are looking at.

syntax: Knowledge of grammar and word associations to make sense of a sentence.

transient channels: A short duration response that shuts off the visual processing of the sustained system. It is triggered by our eye movement when we move our eyes from fixation point to fixation point during reading.

vestibular system: The non-auditory organs of the inner ear dedicated to posture, equilibrium, balance, muscular tones and orientation in environmental space.

vision: Includes not only seeing the 20/20 line of print but all visual skills including focusing, eye teaming and eye tracking.

visual motor: Pertains to eye-hand coordination skills (i.e., the ability to copy and reproduce a geometric shape or letter accurately).

visual motor control (VMC) bat: This is a dowel rod about three feet long and one inch in diameter. It is divided into colored sections and is used for gross motor and eye-hand coordination activities.

visual persistence: Refers to the continued processing of visual information from the previous fixation. it is usually the result of not having the transient channels functioning properly.

walking rail: A 6 to 8 foot long (2 inch x 4 inch) board that is balanced on three (4 inch x 4 inch) sections. It is used for balance and gross motor activities.

Appendices

APPENDIX A: QUESTIONNAIRE

Name: _____   Date:_____

Check the area that best represents the occurrence of each symptom.

Key: N-Never   S-Seldom   O-Occasionally   F-Frequently   A-Always

	N	S	O	F	A

Makes mistakes copying from the board or text
(ET, VMP, Motor, VM)

Loses place easily during reading
(ET, Motor, VM)

Adds or substitutes words during reading
(ET, VM, VMP)

Words appear to run together during reading
(ET, Motor, VM)

Omits or skips words during reading
(ET, Motor, VM)

Complains about having to read and tends to avoid it
(All areas)

Tends to forget what was written on the board or
assignments
(VM, ET, VMP)

Sloppy or disorganized printing or writing
(VMP, ET, Motor)

Needs to have his work modified due to slow reading
(ET, all areas)

Fails to give close attention to details or makes
careless mistakes in schoolwork or other activities
(ET, VM, VMP)

Reverses letters or words
(REV, L,, ET)

Uses his finger to keep his place while reading
(ET, Motor, VMP)

Words appear to jump or move when he reads
(ET, Motor, VMP)

APPENDIX A: QUESTIONNAIRE (CONTINUED)

Key: N-Never   S-Seldom   O-Occasionally   F-Frequently   A-Always

	N	S	O	F	A
Will place letters in the wrong position in words (VMP, ET, REV, LAT)					
Has headaches when he reads (Refer for eye examination.)					
Skips lines when he reads (ET, Motor, VMP)					
Complains of double vision when he reads (Refer for eye examination.)					

APPENDIX B: IMPORTANT NAMES AND ADDRESSES

Kenneth A. Lane, OD, FCOVD
230 W. Main
Lewisville, TX 75057
Telephone: 888-412-LANE
Website: www.lanelearningcenter.com
Email: info@lanelearningcenter.com
Workbooks for visual perceptual activities.

American Optometric Association (AOA)
243 N. Lindbergh Blvd.
St. Louis, MO 63141
Telephone: 314-991-4100
FAX: 314-991-4101
Website: www.aoanet.org
National professional organization for optometrists, reference materials available.

College of Optometrists in Vision Development (COVD)
243 N. Lindbergh Blvd., #310
St. Louis, MO 63141
Telephone: 888-268-3770
FAX: 314-991-1167
Website: www.covd.org
Certifies optometrists in vision development and therapy. Referral for optometrists providing vision therapy and functional vision care.

Optometric Extension Program
1921 E. Carnegie Ave., Suite 3-L
Santa Ana, CA 92705
Telephone: 949.250.8070
FAX: 949.250.8157
Website: www.oep.org
Literature and supplies available.

Parents Active For Vision Education (P.A.V.E.)
4135 54th Place
San Diego, CA 92105
Telephone: 800-PAVE-988
FAX: 619-287-0084
Website: www.pavevision.org
Email: info@pavevision.org
Parent support group for vision education.

The American Occupational Therapy Association, Inc.
4720 Montgomery Lane
P.O. Box 31220
Bethesda, MD 20824-1220
Telephone: 301.652.2682
FAX: 301.652.7711
Website: www.aota.org
The national headquarters of the American Occupational Therapy Association.

Index

Printed in the United States
by Baker & Taylor Publisher Services